MCQs in Medical Virology

MCQs in Medical Virology
A study guide

Steven H. Myint MD, MRCP
Senior Lecturer in Clinical Virology
University of Leicester Medical School
Leicester, UK

and

William L. Irving PhD, MRCPath
Senior Lecturer in Clinical Virology
University of Nottingham Medical School
Nottingham, UK

with a foreword by

Professor J.R. Pattison
Dean of the University College London School of Medicine
London, UK

CHAPMAN & HALL MEDICAL
London · Glasgow · Weinheim · New York · Tokyo · Melbourne · Madras

Published by Chapman & Hall, 2–6 Boundary Row, London SE1 8HN

Chapman & Hall, 2–6 Boundary Row, London SE1 8HN, UK

Blackie Academic & Professional, Wester Cleddens Road, Bishopbriggs, Glasgow G64 2NZ, UK

Chapman & Hall GmbH, Pappelallee 3, 69469 Weinheim, Germany

Chapman & Hall Inc., One Penn Plaza, 41st Floor, New York NY10119, USA

Chapman & Hall Japan, Thomson Publishing Japan, Hirakawacho Nemoto Building, 6F, 1–7–11 Hirakawa-cho, Chiyoda-ku, Tokyo 102, Japan

Chapman & Hall Australia, Thomas Nelson Australia, 102 Dodds Street, South Melbourne, Victoria 3205, Australia

Chapman & Hall India, R. Seshadri, 32 Second Main Road, CIT East, Madras 600 035, India

First edition 1994

© 1994 Steven H. Myint and William L. Irving

Typeset in 10/12pt Times by Mews Photosetting, Beckenham, Kent
Printed in Great Britain by Page Bros, Norwich

ISBN 0 412 47620 7

A catalogue record for this book is available from the British Library

Library of Congress Catalog Card Number 93-74445

∞ Printed on permanent acid-free text paper, manufactured in accordance with the proposed ANSI/NISO Z39.48-1992 and ANSI/NISO Z39.48-1984 (Permanence of Paper).

Contents

Foreword

Developments in medical education and training are taking place throughout the world. A number of themes are common to the changes being considered in various countries and one of these themes concerns the development of a core curriculum with the remainder of the time devoted to options chosen by individual students. There seems little doubt that there would be general agreement to medical virology being an essential part of the core curriculum. Irrespective of where the individual practitioner will end up, either geographically or in terms of specialty choice, there is a requirement to understand the general principles and some of the factual detail of virus diseases. A new study guide is therefore both timely and likely to be of lasting significance. Steven Myint and Will Irving are to be thanked for producing a new medical virology book which I believe will become widely used and run into many editions.

Another of the themes underlying developments in medical education is the need for the development of a good understanding of the general principles early on in education so that a practitioner may apply these to a subject, the details of which will change many times over the succeeding 40 years of practice. At the same time general principles are often best understood and committed to memory with the help of specific examples. Therefore all books must promote the understanding of their subject, be a source of factual information and, we hope, a source of enjoyment to the reader. Steven and Will have chosen to base their study guide on multiple choice questions. As is well known this will be particularly suitable to the requirement to provide factual information. However, each of the chapters in the book is consistently arranged so that there is a commentary on every one of the questions included. This commentary allows the reader to develop an understanding of the subject. Enjoyment is provided by the games-playing element of answering multiple choice questions in the context of developing and understanding of the subject rather than in the usual qualifying examination format.

Devising multiple choice questions is not easy and so the authors are to be congratulated on having produced a comprehensive and consistent guide to the subject of medical virology. The answers to the questions are not all clear-cut and doubtless there will be some for which the answer changes in the course of time. Nevertheless if one is confident enough to argue with the given answer to a question it seems likely that one knows sufficient about the subject to be regarded as an accomplished student. I am in no doubt that the book will be popular with undergraduates and postgraduates alike.

J.R. Pattison

Preface

Medical education in many countries is undergoing change. The amount of material that medical students have been expected to learn has grown exponentially in the last two decades: particularly with the advances in basic medical sciences. This has often been to the detriment of the most important facet of clinical practice: being able to recognize and manage clinical illnesses. Viruses cause the majority of such illnesses and this small book aims to impart practical knowledge regarding the viruses, their clinical manifestations, diagnosis and management. It supplements courses taught to undergraduates and can also be used as a revision text for non-specialists (including general practitioners). The MCQ format promotes active learning, but unlike most books of this genre, detailed coverage is given in the answer section. The questions are designed to probe areas of lack of knowledge and should be used, principally, to learn and not to test.

We are grateful to numerous medical students and trainee micro-biologists on whom these questions have been tested for their comments and criticisms. We must also thank our own teachers and colleagues for helpful discussions. Most of all we are grateful to our long-suffering wives and families who have had to tolerate absentee husbands and fathers.

Both authors have been at University College in London with Professor John Pattison. We hope that we have maintained his high standards and taken virology from the academic 'ivory tower' to the patient's bedside.

Steven H. Myint, Leicester
William L. Irving, Nottingham

How to use this book

This book is a study guide and not a set of examination questions with answers. Thus many questions will test the reader's knowledge in depth and some will be deliberately 'grey'. Nevertheless, we feel that the detailed answers in the book should resolve any ambiguity.

The first half of the book contains questions that are numbered identically to answers set out in the second section. In each section, apart from Paper 1, each paper is similarly oriented. The first few questions or answers are on general aspects of viral infections pertinent to that system, then specific viruses are discussed. There is, usually one question on the virus itself and then questions that cover the clinical manifestations, diagnosis and management of infections caused by that virus. The questions on the biology of the viruses are set in a different typescript, and will be of main interest to undergraduates. Postgraduates, such as MRCP and MRCGP candidates, will find the clinical questions of most relevance.

As the answer section is detailed enough to be used as a source book, the student may wish to read this first and then use the questions to test recall or to highlight gaps in knowledge by doing the questions first. Either way, the tables, in general, are meant to be used if further detail is required and can also be useful 'checklists'. It is hoped that this book may later be a ready and compact reference for clinicians and microbiologists alike.

Questions

Paper 1   Introduction to viruses

1. *Viruses possess the following properties*
(a) *they can replicate in a cell-free environment*
(b) *possess both DNA and RNA*
(c) *may contain their own enzymes*
(d) *always replicate in the cytoplasm of host cells*
(e) *may consist of nucleic acid alone*

2. *The following statements are true in the classification of viruses*
(a) *terms for virus families have the suffix* -**viridae**
(b) *the nature of the genome is a feature used in classification*
(c) *classification of human viruses is different from that of other vertebrate viruses*
(d) *there are over 15 families of viruses that have human pathogens*
(e) *arthropod-borne viruses belong to the virus family* **Arboridae**

3. **The following viruses and routes of infection are matched**
(a) papillomaviruses and genital mucosa
(b) Epstein–Barr virus and respiratory tract
(c) measles virus and the alimentary tract
(d) adenoviruses and the alimentary tract
(e) varicella-zoster virus and the respiratory tract

4. *In the pathogenesis of virus infections, the following statements are true*
(a) *the severity of some virus infections is influenced by host genetic factors*
(b) *with any one virus, the viral load correlates well with the likelihood of disease*
(c) *the age of the host can change the spectrum of disease of any specific virus*
(d) *the presence of pre-existing antibody always protects against infection*
(e) *breastfed infants are less susceptible to infection than infants fed cow's milk*

5. *The following host defence mechanisms are active in the prevention of or recovery from virus infections*
(a) *tears*
(b) *Kupffer cells*
(c) *interferons*
(d) *serum IgG*
(e) *secretory IgA*

6. **Properties of interferons include**
(a) *regulation of cell growth*
(b) *induction by double-stranded RNA*
(c) *prevention of virus replication in infected cells*
(d) *production by all cell types*
(e) *modulation of the immune response*

7. **The effects of viruses at a cellular level include**
(a) *inhibition of cellular protein synthesis*
(b) *transformation*
(c) *cell lysis*
(d) *cell fusion*
(e) *production of inclusion bodies*

8. **The following stages in the replicative cycle of viruses have been exploited as targets by currently licensed antiviral drugs**
(a) *binding to host cell surface receptor*
(b) *transcription of viral nucleic acid*
(c) *packaging of virus*
(d) *virus uncoating*
(e) *viral maturation*

9. **The following are important principles of specimen processing for subsequent viral diagnosis**
(a) specimens are generally best collected at the onset of symptoms
(b) specimens should generally be kept at 37°C for transport to the laboratory
(c) viral transport medium contains antibiotics
(d) specimens should be taken from the site of symptomatic illness for virus culture if possible
(e) paired blood samples should be taken to enable retrospective diagnosis

10. **In the laboratory diagnosis of infection by viruses the following statements are true**
(a) electron microscopy is a more sensitive technique than enzyme-linked immunoassay for the diagnosis of blood-borne viruses.
(b) continuous cell lines are able to support the growth of a broader range of viruses than primary cell strains
(c) the results of a single serum analysed for serum antibodies by complement fixation are never of practical benefit
(d) gene amplification methods are less sensitive than virus culture
(e) haemagglutination-inhibition tests are applicable to the detection of all viruses

11. **The following statements are true**
(a) autoclaving at 121°C for 15 minutes is an effective sterilizing method for virally-contaminated material
(b) immersion in 2% glutaraldehyde for 60 minutes is a reliable means of disinfection of endoscopes contaminated with blood-borne viruses
(c) enveloped viruses are, generally, sensitive to lipid detergents
(d) 70% alcohol is an effective handwashing solution for the reduction of infectivity of rotaviruses
(e) 19% cetrimide is a reliable agent for the disinfection of virally-contaminated surfaces

12. **Patients with the following infections should be routinely isolated**
(a) Lassa fever
(b) herpes simplex
(c) human immunodeficiency virus
(d) rabies
(e) orf

13. **The following are notifiable diseases in the UK**
(a) Lassa fever
(b) rabies
(c) hepatitis B
(d) human immunodeficiency virus
(e) measles

14. Principles of the management and prevention of exposure to blood-borne viruses include
(a) immediate cleaning of wounds after percutaneous injury
(b) rapid reporting systems for accidental exposure
(c) serological testing of the donor if infectious status unknown
(d) the use of double gloves for invasive procedures
(e) vaccination of 'at risk' staff

15. The following statements are true
(a) the risk of transmission of HIV from an infected patient to a healthcare worker (HCW) via a needlestick injury is 0.3%
(b) the risk of transmission of hepatitis B from an infected patient who is HBeAg-positive to a HCW via a needlestick injury is 0.3%
(c) the risk of transmission of hepatitis C from a seropositive patient to a HCW via a needlestick injury is 0.3%
(d) the risk of transmission of HIV from an infected HCW to a patient is 0.3%
(e) the risk of transmission of hepatitis B from an infected HCW to a patient is 0.3%

Paper 2 Viruses and the respiratory tract

1. The following statements are true
- **(a)** bacteria are responsible for 25% of all upper respiratory tract infections in the UK and USA
- **(b)** the commonest single agent associated with the common cold is the human rhinovirus
- **(c)** non-bacterial causes are responsible for less than 25% of lower respiratory tract infections in adults
- **(d)** mortality from respiratory infections is greater in the developing world than in the developed world because of increased incidence of infection
- **(e)** the transmission of respiratory viruses can occur by fomites

2. The following viruses and diseases are commonly associated
- **(a)** parainfluenza virus type 1 and laryngotracheobronchitis
- **(b)** respiratory syncytial virus and bronchiolitis
- **(c)** toroviruses and the common cold
- **(d)** measles and pneumonia in children
- **(e)** adenovirus type 7 and pharyngoconjunctival fever

3. The following are features of common cold viruses
- **(a)** coronavirus colds have a peak incidence in the winter months
- **(b)** only one rhinovirus serotype tends to circulate in any one year in a specific locality
- **(c)** kissing is an effective means of transmission
- **(d)** excretion of virus may persist for 2 weeks after the symptoms have subsided
- **(e)** re-infection with the same serotype of rhinovirus does not occur

4. The following clinical features occur in over 25% of sufferers of colds
- **(a)** fever
- **(b)** headache
- **(c)** myalgia
- **(d)** pneumonia
- **(e)** cough

5. **The following agents used in the management of common colds have antiviral activity**
(a) antihistamines
(b) aspirin
(c) enviroxime
(d) vitamin C
(e) interferon

6. **Common causes (more than 5% of all cases) of pharyngitis include**
(a) Epstein–Barr virus
(b) rhinoviruses
(c) coronaviruses
(d) bacterial causes
(e) human immunodeficiency viruses

7. **The following are causes of acute laryngitis**
(a) influenza A
(b) rotavirus
(c) adenovirus
(d) coxsackie A21
(e) respiratory syncytial virus

8. *Rhinoviruses*
(a)   are non-enveloped
(b)   acid-stable
(c)   can be differentiated into over 110 serotypes
(d)   utilize at least two host cell proteins as receptors
(e)   replicate using a polyprotein intermediate

9. *Coronaviruses*
(a)   possess a single-stranded RNA genome
(b)   use a nested set of subgenomic mRNAs to produce the virion polypeptides
(c)   have only one serotype worldwide
(d)   have been found in diarrhoeal stools
(e)   have been shown to infect ferrets

10. *Human parainfluenza viruses*
(a) *possess a DNA genome*
(b) *possess an envelope*
(c) *will grow in cell monolayers*
(d) *are divided into four antigenic types*
(e) *are sensitive to the antiviral effects of amantadine*

11. **Clinical features of infection with parainfluenza viruses include**
(a) an incubation period of 2–4 days
(b) frequent reinfection with the same serotype
(c) shedding of virus for 10 days after infection
(d) parotitis
(e) Paget's disease of bone

12. *Respiratory syncytial virus*
(a) *is a member of the* **Paramyxoviridae**
(b) *has only one serotype*
(c) *causes syncytial formation in susceptible cell monolayers*
(d) *remains infectious for several months at room temperature*
(e) *is susceptible* in vitro *to ribavirin*

13. **Recognized clinical features of infection with RSV include**
(a) onset of epidemics in August
(b) pneumonia
(c) endocarditis
(d) meningoencephalitis
(e) reinfections with the same subgroup

14. *Adenoviruses*
(a) *possess an envelope*
(b) *have a DNA genome*
(c) *can be classified into over 40 serotypes*
(d) *cannot be grown on cell monolayers*
(e) *are susceptible to ribavirin*

15. **Adenoviruses have been associated with**
(a) pneumonia
(b) diarrhoea
(c) conjunctivitis
(d) pancreatitis
(e) cystitis

16.   Properties of influenza viruses include
(a)   a genome consisting of six discrete strands of RNA
(b)   an envelope
(c)   classification into three types on the basis of differences in their haemagglutinin
(d)   a cytoplasmic site of replication
(e)   the production of a single protein from each strand of RNA.

17.   The following are features of the epidemiology of infection caused by influenza viruses
(a)   influenza epidemics have only occurred since the beginning of this century
(b)   pandemics generally result from 'antigenic shift' of the virus
(c)   influenza A strains are subtyped on the basis of antigens on the haemagglutinin and neuraminidase proteins
(d)   human influenza viruses only infect humans
(e)   the highest rates of infection occur in the elderly

18.   Clinical features of infection with influenza A virus include
(a)   epidemics occurring in the winter months in the Northern hemisphere
(b)   an incubation period of 18–72 hours
(c)   myalgia occurring in the majority of children
(d)   a less severe illness usually than that due to influenza C
(e)   myoglobinuria

19.   The following statements are true
(a)   influenza viruses can be grown in primary monkey kidney cells
(b)   influenza reinfections occur despite high levels of serum antibody
(c)   amantadine hydrochloride is effective as a prophylactic agent against infection with influenza B
(d)   immunity to influenza A after effective vaccination lasts for at least 10 years
(e)   universal vaccination against influenza A is currently recommended

20.   The following viruses have been shown to cause pneumonia
(a)   measles
(b)   varicella-zoster
(c)   herpes simplex
(d)   Inoue–Melnick virus
(e)   cytomegalovirus

Paper 3 Viruses and the neurological system

1. The following associations are well characterized
(a) varicella-zoster virus and Ramsay–Hunt syndrome
(b) enteroviruses and idiopathic (Bell's) facial palsy
(c) human T cell leukaemia virus type 1 (HTLV-1) and tropical spastic paraparesis
(d) enteroviruses and meningitis
(e) rubella and subacute sclerosing panencephalitis (SSPE)

2. Are the following true or false?
(a) viral meningitis is commonest in the late winter months in the UK and USA
(b) meningitis due to lymphocytic choriomeningitis (LCM) virus has characteristically occurred in the spring
(c) Eastern equine encephalitis is endemic in the Far East
(d) person-to-person transmission of rabies is the commonest route of spread
(e) adenoviruses are the second commonest cause of meningitis in the UK

3. Characteristic features distinguishing viral meningitis from bacterial meningitis are
(a) normal cerebrospinal fluid (CSF) glucose levels
(b) predominance of lymphocytes in CSF
(c) drowsiness
(d) fever
(e) photophobia

4. The following are useful in the specific aetiological diagnosis of viral meningitis
(a) electron microscopy of CSF
(b) culture of CSF in cell monolayers
(c) culture of urine
(d) culture of stools
(e) immunofluorescence of CSF

5.   The following statements are true
(a)   person-to-person transmission is a frequent occurrence in meningitis caused by lymphocytic choriomeningitis (LCM) virus
(b)   respiratory symptoms occur in less than 5% of cases of LCM meningitis
(c)   herpes simplex type 2 (HSV-2) is more commonly associated with aseptic meningitis than herpes simplex type 1 (HSV-1)
(d)   herpes simplex meningitis does not occur without encephalitis
(e)   varicella-zoster virus meningitis has a poor prognosis

6.   The following statements regarding viral causes of encephalitis are true
(a)   parainfectious encephalitis can be induced by varicella-zoster virus
(b)   measles encephalitis rarely occurs in an individual who does not have a rash
(c)   adenoviruses account for over 10% of cases of meningoencephalitis in the temperate climates of the Northern hemisphere
(d)   encephalopathy in HIV infection is always caused by opportunistic pathogens
(e)   enterovirus-associated encephalopathy has a good prognosis

7.   The following are recognized causes of encephalitis
(a)   Coxsackie A5
(b)   adenovirus
(c)   herpes simplex-2
(d)   cytomegalovirus
(e)   measles

8.   *Human enteroviruses*
(a)   *are members of the* **Picornaviridae**
(b)   *include coxsackie, polioviruses and echoviruses*
(c)   *are stable at acid pH*
(d)   *replicate in the intestine*
(c)   *can survive exposure to 60°C*

9.   Disease manifestations of enterovirus infection include
(a)   maculopapular rash
(b)   diarrhoea
(c)   myocarditis
(d)   vesicular rash
(e)   meningitis

10. The following statements regarding enteroviral meningitis are true
(a) 50–80% of all cases of viral meningitis are caused by entero-viruses
(b) poor hygiene is a significant factor in the spread of illness
(c) most cases occur in children under 14 years of age
(d) infection most often occurs in the summer months in temperate climates
(e) long-term sequelae of infection never occur

11. Features of infection with polioviruses include
(a) transmission from small mammals
(b) paralytic poliomyelitis occurring in industrialized countries results most often from vaccine strains
(c) destruction of anterior horn cells in cases of paralytic polio-myelitis
(d) isolation of virus from the CSF in the majority of cases
(e) excretion of virus in the stools of patients for months after illness

12. Mumps virus
(a) has a segmented RNA genome
(b) has only one serotype
(c) is shed in the urine of infected individuals
(d) causes subclinical reinfection
(e) can be transmitted by fomites

13. The following statements are true
(a) the presence of parotitis in a patient with aseptic meningitis is reliably diagnostic of mumps meningitis
(b) CSF abnormalities occur in the majority of patients with mumps parotitis
(c) orchitis complicates mumps infection in children under 10 years of age more often than encephalitis
(d) hearing loss from mumps infection always occurs as a result of mumps encephalitis
(e) mumps meningitis occurs most frequently in the winter months in temperate climates

14.   The following statements regarding herpes simplex encephalitis are true

(a)   herpes simplex encephalitis is the commonest identifiable cause of sporadic viral encephalitis in Europe and North America

(b)   HSV-1 is found more commonly than HSV-2 in adults

(c)   the presence of active orolabial herpes is a useful diagnostic indicator of the cause of encephalitis

(d)   the occipital lobes are predominantly affected

(e)   encephalitis due to HSV-2 in neonates has a worse prognosis than that due to HSV-1

15.   Clinical and diagnostic features of herpes simplex encephalitis include

(a)   the presence of primary genital herpes is a positive diagnostic indicator of encephalitis also being due to herpes simplex

(b)   detectable focal neurological signs occur in the majority

(c)   culture of the CSF is positive in less than 5% of cases

(d)   electroencephalography is a helpful examination

(e)   brain biopsy is always needed to confirm the diagnosis

16.   The following are features of arboviral encephalitis

(a)   diagnosis of the specific aetiological agent cannot be made on clinical grounds

(b)   the viruses can be isolated from the CSF in the majority of cases

(c)   vaccines have not been made available

(d)   clinical infections occur more commonly in children than adults

(e)   epidemics are rare

17.   *Rabies virus*

(a)   is enveloped

(b)   is bullet-shaped

(c)   is rapidly inactivated at 60°C

(d)   can be transmitted to humans from cats

(e)   causes the formation of Negri bodies in infected cells

18.   Clinical features of rabies virus infection include

(a)   an incubation period of up to a year

(b)   aggressive behaviour

(c)   hydrophobia

(d)   a poor prognosis in the majority of symptomatic patients

(e)   diagnosis by culture of the virus from the CSF

19. Current rabies vaccines
(a) can be successfully used to control animal reservoirs
(b) are live attenuated strains
(c) have a high frequency of neurological side-effects
(d) must be inoculated into the site of bite from an animal
(e) result in protective antibody in less than 50% of those given post-exposure prophylaxis

20. The following chronic degenerative disorders of the nervous system are thought to have a viral aetiology
(a) Kuru
(b) Creutzfeld–Jacob disease
(c) Parkinson's disease
(d) encephalitis lethargica
(e) Alzheimer's disease

21. Features of subacute sclerosing panencephalitis (SSPE) include
(a) occurrence in Caucasian males more often than African females
(b) a mean incubation period of 25 years
(c) measles virus is detectable in the brain of affected patients
(d) 50% of those affected are over 50 years of age
(e) the majority of patients die within 3 years of onset

22. The following viruses are associated with retinopathy
(a) cytomegalovirus
(b) rubella
(c) rhinovirus
(d) measles
(e) herpes simplex type 1

23. Deafness is associated with the following viruses
(a) hepatitis B
(b) rubella
(c) cytomegalovirus
(d) measles
(e) mumps

24. The following viruses are associated with myopathy
(a) influenza B
(b) Tacaribe
(c) Coxsackie B
(d) Ross River
(e) rhinovirus

25.   The following statements pertaining to chronic fatigue syndrome are true

(a)   fatigue lasting 6 months or more is part of the accepted case definition

(b)   fatigue lasting 6 months or more occurs in less than 1% of the population in industrialized countries

(c)   persistent Epstein–Barr virus infection is the likely common aetiology

(d)   specific diagnostic tests are available

(e)   hypogammaglobulinaemia always occurs

26.   The following statements are true

(a)   neurological abnormalities may occur as a result of infection with Epstein–Barr virus

(b)   Reye's syndrome occurring with influenzal illness in children is associated with the concurrent administration of salicylates

(c)   progressive multifocal leucoencephalopathy is associated with human papillomavirus infection of the brain

(d)   multiple sclerosis is strongly associated with infection of the brain with coronaviruses

(e)   viruses have not been isolated from the CSF of patients with Guillain–Barré syndrome

Paper 4 Viruses and the gastrointestinal tract

1. In temperate climates of the Northern hemisphere
(a) viruses causing gastroenteritis have their highest attack rates in the elderly
(b) most deaths from virus-induced gastroenteritis occur in the elderly
(c) viral-associated gastroenteritis is responsible for less than 10% of total hospital admissions with gastroenteritis
(d) persistent diarrhoea of greater than 14 days duration occurs in over 15% of cases of viral gastroenteritis
(e) persistent diarrhoea is less common than in developing countries

2. Viruses that are implicated in causing acute diarrhoeal illness include
(a) Norwalk virus
(b) astrovirus
(c) enterovirus
(d) rotavirus
(e) hepatitis E

3. The following are useful in the management of an individual with viral gastroenteritis
(a) glucose solutions
(b) rice feeds
(c) antibiotics
(d) breastfeeding
(e) bismuth subsalicylate

4. Principles of the control and prevention of nosocomial outbreaks caused by viral gastrointestinal pathogens include
(a) screening of asymptomatic staff
(b) closure of wards to new admissions until 72 hours after the last case
(c) handwashing after contact with the patient
(d) exclusion of symptomatic staff from work for 48 hours after recovery
(e) exclusion of high-risk foods from food preparation areas

5.   Rotaviruses
(a)   *possess a lipid envelope*
(b)   *possess a segmented genome*
(c)   *replicate in the cytoplasm of enterocytes*
(d)   *that cause infections in humans are serologically identical*
(e)   *are sensitive to lipid detergents*

6.   Features of the epidemiology of rotavirus infections include
(a)   peak incidence of infections due to group A rotaviruses occur in children under 3 months of age
(b)   illness caused by rotaviruses is less likely to result in hospitalization than other viral gastroenteridites
(c)   adults with rotavirus infection tend to have more severe illness than infants
(d)   spread is predominantly by the respiratory route
(e)   infections occur most frequently in the summer months in temperate climates

7.   The clinical spectrum of illness with rotaviruses include
(a)   fever greater than 38.5°C
(b)   watery diarrhoea
(c)   an incubation period of 5–7 days
(d)   tenesmus
(e)   viral meningitis

8.   The following statements regarding rotavirus infection are true
(a)   the immune response to rotavirus infection is predominantly serotype-specific
(b)   reinfections do not occur
(c)   diagnosis of infection is routinely made by culture of the virus in cell monolayers
(d)   management of cases with oral rehydration solutions alone is effective in the majority of cases
(e)   animal strains can induce neutralizing antibodies against human strains

9.   Features of illness due to enteric adenoviruses include
(a)   watery diarrhoea
(b)   preponderance of illness during the winter months
(c)   an incubation period of 2–4 days
(d)   concurrent respiratory tract infection in the majority of cases
(e)   frequent clinical reinfections

10. **The following statements concerning the diagnosis and management of diarrhoeal illness caused by enteric adenoviruses are true**
(a) diagnosis is best made by growth in cell culture
(b) analysis of viral DNA is useful for typing purposes
(c) in cases with respiratory symptoms the virus can be detected in respiratory secretions
(d) ribavirin is useful in reducing the duration of infection
(e) vaccines are available

11. *The following are properties of caliciviruses*
(a) *an envelope*
(b) *a single structural protein*
(c) *a single strand of RNA*
(d) *a capsid with icosahedral symmetry*
(e) *a replication strategy identical to that of enteroviruses*

12. **Disease caused by human enteric caliciviruses of characteristic morphology**
(a) occurs commonly in both children and adults
(b) lasts 1–11 days
(c) is frequently epidemic
(d) is frequently associated with vomiting
(e) can be diagnosed by electron microscopy of stools

13. **The following are features of the epidemiology of disease due to Norwalk and Norwalk-like viruses**
(a) the disease is restricted to Norwalk, Ohio, USA
(b) they are the single most commonly identified agents found as the cause of outbreaks of diarrhoeal disease on cruise ships
(c) the disease predominantly occurs in the summer in temperate climates
(d) spread is most commonly by the respiratory route
(e) the disease predominantly occurs in young adults

14. **Characteristic features of illness due to Norwalk virus are**
(a) vomiting
(b) headache
(c) an illness that lasts 24–48 hours
(d) an incubation period of 12–48 hours
(e) jaundice

15.   Astroviruses
(a)   are only found in humans
(b)   contain a single major polypeptide
(c)   contain an RNA genome
(d)   can be grown in cell culture
(e)   have a characteristic 'star' morphology

16.   Prominent features of illness caused by astroviruses include
(a)   meningitis
(b)   peak incidence in the winter months
(c)   a predilection for young adults
(d)   an incubation period of 5–7 days
(e)   bloody diarrhoea

Paper 5 Viruses and the hepatobiliary tract

1. **Viral hepatitis**
(a) is less frequent than hepatitis caused by other infectious agents
(b) is caused by one of five agents only
(c) due to hepatitis B can usually be distinguished clinically and pathologically from that due to hepatitis A
(d) is most commonly due to hepatitis B in industrialized countries
(e) is rare in the South Pacific Islands

2. **The following viruses have been associated with pancreatitis**
(a) mumps
(b) measles
(c) Coxsackie B4
(d) cytomegalovirus
(e) Tataguine

3. *Features of the hepatitis A virus include*
(a) *a single-stranded RNA genome*
(b) *more than one genotype*
(c) *more than one serotype*
(d) *greater resistance to heat and acid than other members of the* **Picornaviridae**
(e) *inability to grow in cell culture*

4. **Regarding the epidemiology of hepatitis A virus infection**
(a) the majority of infections in developing countries occur in children
(b) the majority of infections in developed countries occur in children
(c) transmission is via the faecal–oral route
(d) outbreaks have commonly been associated with the ingestion of shellfish
(e) infection is more common among male homosexuals than the general population

5.   Clinical features of infection caused by hepatitis A include
(a)   an incubation period of 2–6 weeks
(b)   icteric infection occurring in less than 10% of children under 6 years of age
(c)   serum sickness
(d)   fulminant hepatitis
(e)   increased severity of illness in pregnant women in the USA

6.   The diagnosis of infection due to recent or current hepatitis A infection
(a)   can usually be made by the detection of hepatitis A IgM at the onset of clinical illness
(b)   can usually be made by the detection of hepatitis A IgM 3 months after the onset of clinical illness
(c)   can be made by the detection of hepatitis A in stools during the first week of illness
(d)   can reliably be made by the detection of virus-specific IgA in saliva during the first week of illness
(e)   can reliably be made by culture of the virus from blood during the first week of illness

7.   The following are useful in the management of infection with hepatitis A
(a)   routine hospitalization of cases
(b)   routine isolation of cases
(c)   prophylaxis with human normal immunoglobulin of kitchen employees in contact with an index case
(d)   routine prophylaxis with human normal immunoglobulin of travellers from Sweden to Greece
(e)   cooking of all shellfish from natural waters prior to consumption

8.   The following statements regarding the HM175 hepatitis A vaccine are true
(a)   it is inactivated
(b)   parenteral administration of vaccine results in lower levels of serum antibody than natural infection
(c)   the concurrent use of human immunoglobulin is contraindicated
(d)   it is recommended in the UK that sewerage workers are routinely vaccinated
(e)   adverse effects are reported in over 10% of vaccinees

9. *Hepatitis B virus*
(a) *is a member of the* **Picornaviridae**
(b) *produces an excess of surface protein when replicating in liver cells*
(c) *can be classified into subtypes on the basis of antigenic differences in the surface antigen*
(d) *possesses a reverse transcriptase*
(e) *possesses a gene which produces a cancer-inducing product*

10. Features of the epidemiology of hepatitis B include
(a) a higher prevalence in industrialized than developing countries
(b) country to country variation of predominant antigenic subtypes
(c) a declining incidence in developed countries
(d) higher prevalence in injectable drug users than the general population
(e) higher prevalence in homosexual than heterosexual men

11. In clinical illness caused by hepatitis B virus
(a) the incubation period prior to jaundice is 2–6 months
(b) HBsAg cannot be detected in the blood for 2–6 months after infection
(c) maculopapular rashes occur
(d) fewer than 10% are anicteric
(e) over 99% of icteric cases resolve completely

12. Evidence for the role of hepatitis B virus in causing primary hepatocellular carcinoma (PHC) includes
(a) higher seroprevalence of HBsAg in patients with PHC than in the general population
(b) higher seroprevalence of HBsAg in patients with PHC than in patients with other malignancies
(c) higher prevalence of PHC in HBsAg carriers than the general population
(d) the development of PHC can be experimentally induced by hepatitis B virus infection of marmosets
(e) the presence of detectable HBsAg in all cases of PHC

13. The following statements regarding serological tests of hepatitis B infection are true
(a) HBsAg can usually be detected before the onset of jaundice
(b) the presence of anti-HBe antibody is a measure of greater infectivity
(c) the presence of anti-HBc IgM indicates current or recent acute infection
(d) anti-HBs is usually detectable before the loss of HBsAg
(e) 100% of patients develop anti-HBs after natural infection

14.   The following statements regarding the management of infection with hepatitis B virus are true

(a)   dextrose infusions are useful in the management of fulminant hepatitis

(b)   acyclovir has been shown to be useful in the treatment of acute hepatitis B

(c)   chronic hepatitis B infection in heterosexual men responds more favourably to arabinoside-A than chronic hepatitis B infection in homosexual men

(d)   alpha-interferon has been shown to be superior to beta-interferon in inducing a favourable clinical response

(e)   chronic hepatitis B acquired in childhood responds more favourably to interferon therapy than chronic hepatitis B acquired in adulthood

15.   Prevention of hepatitis B infection is facilitated by

(a)   the use of genetically engineered vaccines

(b)   the use of hepatitis B immunoglobulin (HBIG) 2 weeks after high risk exposure

(c)   vaccination of all babies born to HBeAg-positive mothers

(d)   testing for anti-HBs titres post-vaccination in the immuno-compromised

(e)   routine booster doses of vaccine annually

16.   Risk factors for non-response to current hepatitis B vaccines include

(a)   obesity

(b)   previous natural infection with hepatitis B virus

(c)   previous infection with hepatitis A virus

(d)   being of female sex

(e)   being immunocompromised

17.   *Hepatitis C*

(a)   *is structurally related to flaviviruses*

(b)   *is the commonest cause of post-transfusion hepatitis in the USA*

(c)   *can be cultivated routinely in cell monolayers*

(d)   *can infect chimpanzees*

(e)   *has been implicated as an aetiological factor in the genesis of primary hepatocellular carcinoma*

18. Clinical and diagnostic features of infection with hepatitis C include
(a) an incubation period of 6–9 weeks following blood transfusion
(b) infectivity of blood from patients a week before clinical illness
(c) chronic hepatitis occurring in 5–10%
(d) successful response of chronic hepatitis to alpha-interferon
(e) rapid diagnosis of acute infection by the detection of C100 antibodies

19. Hepatitis D virus
(a) is a togavirus
(b) contains an RNA genome
(c) is transmitted by blood and blood products
(d) is transmitted by penetrative sexual intercourse
(e) is found in over 50% of hepatitis B carriers in southeast Asia

20. Features of co-infection with hepatitis D and B include
(a) increased rate of fulminant hepatitis in patients with acute hepatitis B
(b) biphasic hepatitic illness in 10% of patients
(c) an increased likelihood of patients with chronic hepatitis B carriage
(d) the presence of delta antigen detectable before the onset of clinical illness
(e) prevention of hepatitis B infection in practice preventing illness from hepatitis D

21. Hepatitis E virus
(a) has a single-stranded RNA genome
(b) can be readily grown in cell monolayer culture
(c) has an envelope
(d) is transmitted by the faecal–oral route
(e) is endemic in northern Europe

22. Features of infection with hepatitis E virus include
(a) an incubation period of 30–40 days
(b) 10% mortality in pregnant women
(c) occurrence of clinical infection predominantly in young adults
(d) routine diagnosis by a complement fixation test
(e) risk of chronic liver disease in 10%

Paper 6   Viruses and the mucocutaneous system

1. The following viruses typically cause both an exanthem and an enanthem
(a) measles
(b) papillomavirus
(c) rubella
(d) orf
(e) human parvovirus B19

2. The following viruses and rashes are matched
(a) rubella and maculopapular rash
(b) herpes simplex type 1 and erythema multiforme
(c) varicella-zoster and vesicular rash
(d) orf and nodular rash
(e) human herpesvirus 6 and maculopapular rash

3. Measles virus
(a) is a member of the **Paramyxoviridae**
(b) has only one serotype
(c) is rapidly inactivated by heat
(d) possesses a haemagglutinin protein
(e) possesses a neuraminidase protein

4. The following are features of the epidemiology of measles
(a) seasonal peaks of illness occur between February and April in temperate climates
(b) transmission is via the respiratory tract
(c) only a minority of susceptible individuals are affected in an outbreak
(d) infection in hospitalized children in Africa has a mortality rate in excess of 5%
(e) over 95% of adults in developed countries have antibody to measles

5. Clinical features of measles virus infection include
(a) infectivity before the onset of symptoms
(b) a prodrome with upper respiratory tract symptoms
(c) Koplik's spots usually appearing after the exanthem
(d) illness occurring in vaccinated patients
(e) lifelong immunity to reinfection after natural infection

6. Recognized complications of measles infection include
(a) pneumonia
(b) encephalitis
(c) myocarditis
(d) secondary bacterial infection
(e) thrombocytopenia

7. Aspects of the diagnosis of measles virus infection include
(a) clinical features alone are rarely sufficient to make a diagnosis
(b) virus can be recovered from the rash
(c) virus can be isolated from nasopharyngeal secretions for 2 days after the onset of rash
(d) virus can be isolated from urine for 4 days after the onset of rash
(e) measles-specific IgG is usually detectable in the CSF of patients with acute encephalitis

8. Current measles vaccines
(a) are live attenuated strains
(b) are routinely used in the UK and USA as a triple vaccine with mumps and rubella
(c) can be used for post-exposure prophylaxis
(d) inhibit the cell-mediated immune response to tuberculin
(e) are best administered in childhood

9. *Rubella virus*
(a) is a member of the **Togaviridae**
(b) is arthropod-borne
(c) can be grown in cell culture
(d) possesses a haemagglutinin
(e) is rapidly inactivated at 56°C

10. Features of the epidemiology of infection with rubella virus include
(a) worldwide distribution
(b) peaks of infection in March to May in temperate climates
(c) epidemics occurring every 10–30 years in countries without universal vaccination
(d) transmission occurring in 90% of susceptible individuals who are in close contact with an index case for 5 minutes
(e) clinical illness rarely occurring in adulthood

11.   Clinical features due to rubella
(a)   may be inapparent in 50% of infected children
(b)   include a rash that starts on the face
(c)   include lymphadenopathy in 80% of symptomatic cases
(d)   include arthritis occurring in men more often than women
(e)   include thrombocytopenic purpura in 25% of cases

12.   Features of the congenital rubella syndrome include
(a)   association with primary maternal infection in the first trimester
of pregnancy
(b)   sensorineural deafness
(c)   cataracts
(d)   pulmonary artery stenosis
(e)   diagnosis by detecting rubella-specific IgG in the fetus

13.   The following statements are true
(a)   haemagglutination-inhibition (HAI) is a commonly used test format
to detect rubella-specific antibodies
(b)   single radial haemolysis (SRH) is a useful test for the detection
of rubella-specific IgM antibodies
(c)   patients are considered immune to rubella infection if they
have a serum antibody level measured by SRH of 15 IU/ml or
greater
(d)   rubella-specific IgM is often present at the onset of rash
(e)   rubella-specific IgM rarely persists for more than a month after
natural infection

14.   Current rubella vaccines
(a)   are inactivated
(b)   may cause thrombocytopenia
(c)   may cause arthritis
(d)   result in seroconversion in 95% of vaccines
(e)   should be an indication for termination if given inadvertently during
pregnancy

15.   *Human parvovirus B19*
(a)   is a defective virus
(b)   is enveloped
(c)   contains a DNA genome
(d)   can be readily grown in cell monolayers
(e)   has only a single serotype

16. Regarding the epidemiology of infection due to B19
(a) infection is only recognized in temperate climates
(b) infection is most commonly acquired in the first 2 years of life
(c) in the UK, infections are commoner in the first six months of the year than in the second six months
(d) the incubation period is 2–4 days
(e) transmission is most commonly by blood and blood products

17. Disease manifestations of B19 infections include
(a) erythema infectiosum
(b) arthritis
(c) aplastic crises
(d) purpura
(e) hydrops fetalis

18. The following are features of human herpesvirus-6 (HHV-6)
(a) it has greater gene and antigen relatedness to cytomegalovirus than other herpesviruses
(b) it exhibits lymphotropism
(c) it can be readily grown in cell monolayers
(d) it can be detected in saliva
(e) sexual transmission is the predominant mode of spread

19. Clinical and diagnostic features of HHV-6 infection include
(a) roseola infantum
(b) Kawasaki disease
(c) exanthem subitum
(d) progression of HIV disease
(e) the presence of HHV-6 IgM is completely reliable as an indication of primary infection

20. Varicella-zoster virus (VZV)
(a) is a member of the **Herpesviridae**
(b) possesses a thymidine kinase
(c) has only one serotype
(d) shares antigens with herpes simplex
(e) remains latent in dorsal root ganglia

21. **The following are epidemiological features of infection with VZV**
(a) worldwide distribution
(b) peak incidence in the winter and early spring in temperate climates
(c) peak incidence in children under 2 years of age in temperate climates
(d) over 95% of young adults in temperate climates are seropositive
(e) over 95% of young adults in tropical countries are seropositive

22. **Characteristic clinical features of chickenpox include**
(a) infectivity before the onset of rash
(b) incubation period of 10–21 days
(c) vesicular rash that starts on the trunk
(d) higher rate of pneumonia in the immunocompromised
(e) lifelong immunity to VZV-induced disease following primary infection

23. **Recognized features of herpes zoster include**
(a) a prodrome lasting weeks
(b) urinary retention
(c) lymphadenitis
(d) occurrence in children
(e) increased frequency in patients with malignancy

24. **The following statements regarding the diagnosis of VZV infection are true**
(a) most cases of VZV infection require laboratory confirmation
(b) virus can be isolated from vesicles in both chickenpox and herpes zoster
(c) virus usually causes cytopathic effects in cell culture in 48–72 hours
(d) a single high titre of specific antibody detectable by CFT may indicate recent infection
(e) screening of healthcare workers who do not have a history of chickenpox is unhelpful because 95% will be seronegative

25. **The following have been shown to be potentially useful in the management and prevention of diseases caused by VZV**
(a) acyclovir
(b) zoster immune globulin
(c) capsaicin
(d) OKA vaccine
(e) acupuncture

26. *The following are features of poxviruses*
(a) *they possess an envelope*
(b) *they possess an RNA genome*
(c) *they replicate entirely in the cytoplasm of infected cells*
(d) *they all have non-primate hosts*
(e) *they can all be grown routinely in cell monolayers*

27. **Are the following statements true or false?**
(a) cowpox produces vesicular lesions on the face
(b) orf and pseudocowpox produce identical clinical lesions
(c) monkeypox usually affects the elderly
(d) reinfections with orf are rare
(e) tanapox classically causes multiple nodular lesions on the face

28. **The following statements are true**
(a) Kawasaki disease is caused by coxsackie B16
(b) Q fever is due to adenovirus type 4
(c) squamous cell carcinoma can result from infection of the skin with human papillomaviruses
(d) eczema vaccinatum is a result of disseminated herpes simplex skin infection
(e) rash only occurs in cases of infectious mononucleosis after the administration of ampicillin

Paper 7   Viruses and the genitourinary tract

1.   Sexual transmission is a documented feature of the following viruses
(a)   hepatitis B
(b)   coronavirus OC43
(c)   human immunodeficiency virus type 1
(d)   human papillomavirus type 6
(e)   Marburg virus

2.   The following diseases and viruses are matched
(a)   urethritis and adenovirus type 37
(b)   genital ulceration and herpes simplex type 1
(c)   genital wart and Epstein–Barr virus
(d)   haemorrhagic cystitis and adenovirus type 11
(e)   glomerulonephritis and hepatitis B

3.   General properties of herpesviruses include
(a)   a double-stranded DNA genome
(b)   an icosahedral capsid
(c)   a tegument
(d)   an envelope
(e)   resistance to lipid detergents

4.   Features of the epidemiology of herpes simplex virus infections include
(a)   herpes simplex type 2 (HSV-2) infection is uncommon before puberty
(b)   herpes simplex type 1 (HSV-1) is usually acquired during the first decade of life
(c)   transmission occurs most commonly by the respiratory route
(d)   transmission rarely occurs from asymptomatic individuals
(e)   prevalence of HSV-2 antibody is higher in prostitutes than in the general adult population in developed countries

5.   Clinical syndromes due to herpes simplex viruses include
(a) gingivostomatitis
(b) whitlow
(c) encephalitis
(d) keratitis
(e) genital ulceration

6.   The following statements regarding genital herpes infection are true
(a) herpes simplex viruses are the most common cause of genital ulceration in developed countries
(b) the majority are due to HSV-2
(c) patients who have had previous gingivostomatitis caused by HSV-1 have a milder illness with primary genital infection due to HSV-2
(d) symptoms occur 1–2 days after contact
(e) asymptomatic shedding occurs in 1–3% of all women

7.   Characteristic clinical features of anogenital infection caused by herpes simplex viruses include
(a) regional lymphadenopathy in primary attacks
(b) primary attacks due to HSV-2 have a higher recurrence rate than those due to HSV-1
(c) mean time to healing of 30 days in primary infections
(d) recurrent infections are milder and of shorter duration than primary attacks
(e) culture of virus from the cervix is less successful in primary attacks than in recurrent infections

8.   The following statements regarding genital herpes infection in pregnant women are true
(a) recurrent infections are more frequent but not more severe in pregnant than non-pregnant women
(b) primary infection in the first trimester of pregnancy is associated with higher risk of fetal loss than normal
(c) infection of the foetus *in utero* is associated with keratoconjunctivitis at birth
(d) primary maternal infection at term is five times more likely to result in neonatal infection than recurrent maternal infection at term
(e) more than 50% of mothers of infants with neonatal infection have a history of previous or current genital herpes

9. **Clinical features of neonatal HSV infection include**
(a) asymptomatic infection in the majority
(b) encephalitis with a poorer prognosis if due to HSV-2 than HSV-1
(c) the occurrence of disseminated infection in the absence of skin lesions
(d) absence of mortality with acyclovir therapy
(e) 50% mortality in untreated patients with localized oral disease

10. **The following measures are cost-effective in the prevention of neonatal infection in developed countries**
(a) delivery of all pregnant women with a history of genital herpes by caesarean section
(b) weekly screening of pregnant women for genital infection from week 34 until term
(c) careful vaginal examination at term
(d) acyclovir prophylaxis given at term to women with a history of herpes genitalis
(e) daily examination of the 'high-risk' neonate for a month after delivery

11. **The following techniques are applied to differentiate HSV-1 from HSV-2**
(a) electron microscopy
(b) immunofluorescence
(c) culture in cell monolayers
(d) genetic analysis of viral DNA
(e) antigen detection by ELISA

12. **The following statements regarding the management and prevention of HSV infection are true**
(a) acyclovir treatment eradicates latent virus
(b) HSV-2 induced neonatal disease is more resistant to treatment with acyclovir than HSV-1 disease
(c) oral acyclovir is useful as a suppressive agent in patients with recurrent genital herpes
(d) the use of topical 5% acyclovir shortens the duration of recurrent attacks of genital herpes
(e) topical surfactant reduces the time of shedding of primary genital herpes

13. ***Molluscum contagiosum virus***
(a) *is a poxvirus*
(b) *is routinely cultivable in cell monolayers*
(c) *has two recognized subtypes*
(d) *usually causes lesions on the trunk and face in children*
(e) *is transmitted by direct skin inoculation*

14. Features of infection caused by molluscum contagiosum include
(a) multiple lesions, typically
(b) characteristic umbilication of lesions
(c) conjunctivitis
(d) spontaneous resolution that normally takes a year
(e) successful treatment with podophyllin

15. ***Human papillomaviruses***
(a) *are members of the* **Poxviridae**
(b) *have serological cross-reactivity with polyomaviruses*
(c) *are typed into over 60 serotypes*
(d) *are tropic for epithelial cells*
(e) *can integrate into human chromosomes*

16. Epidemiological features of human papillomaviruses include
(a) transmission by fomites
(b) transmission by sexual activity
(c) the majority of infections are subclinical
(d) 90% of adolescents in developed countries have had clinically evident cutaneous warts due to papillomaviruses
(e) genital infection with human papillomaviruses is transmitted to fewer than 10% of sexual contacts of an index case

17. Clinical manifestations of human papillomavirus (HPV) infection include
(a) laryngeal papillomatosis
(b) cervical intra-epithelial neoplasia
(c) condyloma lata
(d) squamous cell carcinoma
(e) oral papillomatosis

18.   The following are associated with human papillomavirus infection of the genital tract

(a)   condyloma acuminata
(b)   acetowhite lesions
(c)   vulval carcinoma
(d)   cervical carcinoma
(e)   Buschke–Lowenstein tumour

19.   Recognized risk factors in the development of genital cancer include

(a)   previous HSV-2 infection
(b)   HPV-16 infection
(c)   cigarette smoking
(d)   chronic exposure to sunlight
(e)   oral contraceptive use

20.   The following are useful in the diagnosis of HPV infections

(a)   cervical cytology
(b)   culture of cervical mucus in cell monolayers
(c)   Southern blotting of HPV DNA
(d)   colposcopy
(e)   iodine staining

21.   Agents that have been useful in the management of HPV infection include

(a)   podophyllin
(b)   podophyllotoxin
(c)   salicylate paste
(d)   liquid nitrogen
(e)   alpha-interferon

Paper 8   Retroviruses and AIDS

1.   *The following are features of the retrovirus family*
(a)   *all retroviruses contain the enzyme reverse transcriptase*
(b)   *humans and primates are the only known species to be infected by retroviruses*
(c)   *retroviruses possess a double-stranded DNA genome*
(d)   *retroviruses possess a lipid envelope*
(e)   *some retrovirus genomes contain oncogenes*

2.   *Which of the following viruses are human retroviruses?*
(a)   *human B cell lymphotropic virus*
(b)   *human foamy virus*
(c)   *human T cell lymphotropic virus types 1 and 2*
(d)   *JC and BK viruses*
(e)   *simian immunodeficiency virus (SIV)*

3.   **Regarding human T lymphotropic virus (HTLV-1)**
(a)   seroprevalence studies indicate that infection with this virus is evenly spread throughout the world
(b)   the CD4 molecule acts as a receptor on susceptible cells
(c)   infection is a risk factor for the development of tropical spastic paraparesis
(d)   it may be a cofactor in accelerating the progression of HIV-mediated disease
(e)   it is linked with the pathogenesis of hairy cell leukaemia

4.   **The following are at risk of acquiring HTLV-1 infection**
(a)   recipients of blood transfusions
(b)   sexual partners of HTLV-1 infected individuals
(c)   babies of HTLV-1 infected mothers
(d)   haemophiliacs receiving factor VIII concentrate or cryoprecipitate
(e)   intravenous drug abusers

5. Regarding adult T cell leukaemia/lymphoma (ATLL)
(a) lymphomatous infiltration of the skin may be the presenting feature
(b) the lifetime risk of development of ATLL in an individual known to be anti-HTLV-1 positive is of the order of 50%
(c) DNA copies of the HTLV-1 genome are found in the malignant cells
(d) is associated with hypercalcaemia
(e) first-line therapy consists of azidothymidine

6. Regarding tropical spastic paraparesis (TSP)
(a) the mean age at onset is usually in young adults (15–25 years)
(b) characteristic presentation is with an acute episode of paralysis followed by remissions and acute relapses
(c) it occurs only in Japan and the Caribbean
(d) the CSF contains antibody to HTLV-1
(e) treatment with high-dose steroids results in cessation of disease progression

7. HTLV-II infection
(a) has not been described in the UK
(b) may result in neurological disease similar to HTLV-1 associated myelopathy (HAM)
(c) is diagnosed by demonstrating the presence of antibodies in patients sera
(d) can be transmitted by needle-sharing intravenous drug abusers
(e) occurs in CD8-positive T cells

8. *The human immunodeficiency virus type 1 (HIV-1) genome encodes which of the following proteins*
(a) *a DNA integrase enzyme*
(b) *a protease enzyme which breaks down the polyproteins resulting from RNA translation*
(c) *glycosylating enzymes which glycosylate the surface glycoproteins of the virus*
(d) *the v-myc oncogene*
(e) *several regulatory proteins which control HIV replication*

9. **Which of the following statements relating to the HIV replication cycle are correct?**
(a) the CD8 molecule acts as a receptor for the virus
(b) HIV isolates differ in their cellular tropism in vitro
(c) reverse transcription of the RNA genome of HIV results in an exact double-stranded DNA copy of the virus
(d) once inside a cell the RNA genome of HIV can exist in a latent form free in the cytoplasm
(e) HIV is better able to replicate in a resting T cell than in an activated one

10. **The following are recognized routes of transmission of HIV**
(a) blood transfusion
(b) heterosexual intercourse
(c) breastfeeding
(d) droplet spread
(e) heat-treated factor VIII

11. **Mother-to-baby transmission**
(a) is more likely to occur in mothers who have AIDS than in asymptomatic anti-HIV positive mothers
(b) occurs in over 50% of infants born to HIV carrier mothers
(c) is diagnosed by demonstrating the presence of anti-HIV in blood taken from the neonate within a few days of birth
(d) may occur *in utero* intra-partum or postnatally
(e) results in death in the first year of life of over 90% of the HIV-infected offspring

12. **Regarding accidental transmission of HIV**
(a) the risk of infection following a needlestick injury derived from a known anti-HIV-positive patient is of the order of 10%
(b) splashing of HIV-positive blood onto intact skin may result in transmission of infection
(c) a 6-week course of azidothymidine (60 mg/day) will prevent needlestick transmission of infection provided the course is begun within 24 hours of exposure
(d) HIV can survive and remain infectious in dried blood spilt onto an inanimate surface for up to 7 days
(e) hypochlorite or glutaraldehyde are suitable agents for disinfecting instruments or surfaces contaminated with HIV-positive blood

13.   The following statements regarding the laboratory diagnosis of HIV infection are true

(a)   a negative anti-HIV result is proof that the patient is not infected with HIV

(b)   culture of HIV from the patient's peripheral blood is a reliable diagnostic strategy

(c)   the 'window period' between the time of infection and the generation of detectable anti-HIV can be of the order of 3 months

(d)   p24 antigen testing is a reliable alternative diagnostic approach during the window period

(e)   testing should only be performed with the consent of the patient after appropriate counselling

14.   The following statements relating to acute HIV seroconverting illness are true

(a)   it occurs in the majority of patients

(b)   the commonest presentation is with a glandular fever-like syndrome

(c)   anti-HIV antibody is detectable at the time of this illness

(d)   patients who present with a seroconverting illness have a worse prognosis than those who undergo asymptomatic seroconversion

(e)   patients are not infectious at this stage of their HIV infection

15.   The following are 'AIDS-defining' illnesses in an HIV-positive individual

(a)   herpes zoster

(b)   Kaposi's sarcoma

(c)   oral candidiasis

(d)   oral hairy leukoplakia

(e)   *Pneumocystis carinii* pneumonia

16.   *The following mechanisms may underlie the immunodeficiency associated with HIV infection*

(a)   *virus-induced lysis of CD4-positive cells*

(b)   *cytotoxic T cell destruction of CD4-positive cells*

(c)   *antibody-dependent cellular cytotoxicity directed against uninfected CD4-positive cells to which gp120 has bound*

(d)   *impairment of macrophage/monocyte function by HIV infection*

(e)   *destruction of follicular dendritic cells within lymph nodes*

17. The following are recognized manifestations of AIDS
(a) Burkitt's lymphoma
(b) cerebral toxoplasmosis
(c) nasopharyngeal carcinoma
(d) cytomegalovirus colitis
(e) progressive multifocal leucoencephalopathy

18. Which of the following statements are true?
(a) the diagnosis of *Pneumocystls curinii* pneumonia (PCP) can easily be made on a routine sputum sample
(b) cerebral toxoplasmosis is easily diagnosed by demonstrating a rise in anti-toxoplasma antibodies
(c) cryptococcal meningitis is diagnosed by Gram staining of cerebrospinal fluid
(d) the diagnosis of infection with *Mycobacterium avium-intracellulare complex (MAC)* can be made by culture of the organisms from blood
(e) patients who recover from PCP are still at risk of further attacks

19. HIV-2
(a) is more similar at the genome level to SIV than it is to HIV-1
(b) accounts for the majority of HIV-associated disease in the Gambia and other West African countries
(c) anti-HIV-2 antibody positive blood donors will be reliably identified by the diagnostic assays currently used to screen donors for anti-HIV-1
(d) the rate of progression of HIV-2 infection to AIDS is the same as for HIV-1 infection
(e) has not been described in the UK

20. The following drugs are reverse transcriptase inhibitors
(a) ribavirin
(b) dideoxyinosine
(c) azidothymidine (AZT)
(d) zalcitabine
(e) interferon-alpha

21.   Which of the following statements relating to AZT are true?

(a)   treatment of patients with AIDS results in increased CD4 counts and decreased p24 antigen levels

(b)   treatment of asymptomatic anti-HIV-positive patients delays the onset of AIDS and improves long-term survival

(c)   combination of AZT with acyclovir results in improved survival

(d)   AZT therapy should be continued while patients are taking ganciclovir

(e)   resistance to AZT develops invariably in patients taking the drug for at least 6 months

Paper 9 Tropical viruses

1.   The following viruses and endemic areas are matched
(a)   yellow fever and southeast Asia
(b)   dengue and East Africa
(c)   Lassa fever and West Africa
(d)   Sindbis and northern Europe
(e)   Ross River and Australia

2.   Causes of viral haemorrhagic fever include
(a)   Lassa fever virus
(b)   Marburg virus
(c)   dengue virus
(d)   O'nyong nyong virus
(e)   yellow fever virus

3.   Clinical features of viral haemorrhagic fever include
(a)   lymphopenia
(b)   frank bleeding
(c)   proteinuria
(d)   platelet dysfunction
(e)   hypovolaemic shock

**4.   The following statements regarding the diagnosis and manage-
        ment of viral haemorrhagic fever are true**
(a)   person-to-person transmission is uncommon
(b)   isolation of all cases is recommended
(c)   specimens from patients suspected of being infected should
      not be sent to the laboratory without prior discussion with the
      laboratory
(d)   most cases are diagnosed by culture of virus from the blood of
      the patient
(e)   ribavirin is useful for the treatment of Lassa fever

Paper 10 Miscellaneous viruses and syndromes

1. Epstein–Barr virus (EBV)
(a) is rarely found in tropical countries
(b) is a herpesvirus
(c) can become latent in B lymphocytes
(d) can cause cell transformation
(e) is transmitted predominantly by saliva

2. Diseases associated with EBV infection include
(a) acute infectious mononucleosis
(b) aplastic anaemia
(c) X-linked lymphoproliferative syndrome
(d) non-endemic Burkitt's lymphoma
(e) transplant-associated lymphoproliferative syndrome

3. Features of infectious mononucleosis due to EBV include
(a) an incubation period of 7–14 days
(b) sore throat
(c) fever
(d) jaundice
(e) lymphadenopathy

4. Recognized complications of infectious mononucleosis include
(a) depression
(b) cranial nerve palsies
(c) splenic rupture
(d) pneumonia
(e) orchitis

5. The following are useful in the diagnosis of infection with EBV
(a) detection of cold agglutinins
(b) Paul–Bunnell test
(c) Monospot test
(d) detection of antibody to capsid antigens
(e) detection of antibody to nuclear antigens

6. **The following drugs are indicated in the management of EBV-associated disease**
- **(a)** acyclovir
- **(b)** alpha-interferon
- **(c)** anti-B lymphocyte monoclonal antibodies
- **(d)** ribavirin
- **(e)** metronidazole

7. **Cytomegalovirus (CMV)**
- **(a)** causes cell swelling in susceptible cell monolayers
- **(b)** exhibits latency
- **(c)** exhibits antigenic diversity
- **(d)** is most frequently acquired in the first year of life in both developed and developing countries
- **(e)** can be transmitted by blood and blood products

8. **Recognized clinical features of infection with CMV in adults include**
- **(a)** an incubation period of 1–2 months
- **(b)** infectious mononucleosis
- **(c)** peripheral neuropathy
- **(d)** pneumonia
- **(e)** haemolytic anaemia

9. **Features of neonatal infection with CMV**
- **(a)** presentation may be several weeks after birth
- **(b)** 30% mortality in babies with overt disease at birth
- **(c)** hepatosplenomegaly
- **(d)** hydrops fetalis
- **(e)** microcephaly

10. **The diagnosis of active infection with CMV can be confirmed by**
- **(a)** culture of urine
- **(b)** a single high titre of anti-CMV antibody detected by complement fixation
- **(c)** detection of viral antigens in bronchoalveolar lavage material
- **(d)** electron microscopy of urine
- **(e)** the presence of 'owl's eye' intranuclear inclusions in bronchoalveolar lavage material

11. The following have been used in the management and prevention of infection with CMV
(a) ganciclovir prophylaxis of renal transplant patients
(b) administration of CMV seronegative blood only to CMV seronegative transplant recipients
(c) vaccination with the Towne strain
(d) ganciclovir treatment of chorioretinitis
(e) regular surveillance for CMV infection in the immunocompromised

12. The following malignancies are thought to have a viral aetiology
(a) primary hepatocellular carcinoma
(b) colonic carcinoma
(c) adult T cell leukaemia
(d) African Burkitt's lymphoma
(e) mesothelioma

13. Screening for antibody to the following viruses is useful before starting patients with malignancy on chemotherapy
(a) herpes simplex
(b) varicella-zoster
(c) measles
(d) hepatitis B
(e) parainfluenza type 1

14. The following viruses are associated with aplastic anaemia
(a) human parvovirus B19
(b) Epstein–Barr virus
(c) cytomegalovirus
(d) herpes simplex type 1
(e) dengue

15. Thrombocytopenia has been associated with infection by
(a) human parvovirus B19
(b) rhinovirus
(c) Epstein–Barr virus
(d) varicella-zoster virus
(e) measles virus

16. The following viruses are associated with congenital abnormalities
(a) cytomegalovirus
(b) rubella
(c) herpes simplex type 1
(d) human parvovirus B19
(e) varicella-zoster virus

17. The following statements regarding viral conjunctivitis are true
(a) over 10% of cases of conjunctivitis in adults are due to viruses
(b) over 10% of cases of conjunctivitis in children are due to viruses
(c) herpes simplex type 1 is the commonest single cause of non-epidemic conjunctivitis in young children
(d) adenoviruses are the commonest cause of epidemic conjunctivitis in developed countries
(e) the discharge in cases of viral conjunctivitis is usually purulent

18. Keratitis
(a) may result from infection with herpes simplex type 2
(b) due to herpes simplex type 1 recurs in over 25% of cases
(c) due to adenovirus in epidemic keratoconjunctivitis responds well to topical corticosteroids
(d) occurs in 10% of patients with facial nerve lesions due to varicella-zoster virus
(e) due to measles rarely causes blindness in the UK

19. Myocarditis has been associated with
(a) hepatitis B virus
(b) Coxsackie B virus
(c) Coxsackie A virus
(d) rubella virus
(e) influenza A virus

20. The following viruses have been associated with arthritis
(a) rubella
(b) hepatitis B
(c) mumps
(d) human parvovirus B19
(e) herpes simplex type 1

21. The following viruses and diseases are associated
(a) herpesviruses and atherosclerosis
(b) hepatitis C virus and porphyria cutanea tarda
(c) meningioma and Inoue–Melnick virus
(d) Alzheimer's disease and enteroviruses
(e) vasculitis and cytomegalovirus

22. The following autoantibodies are recognized to result from specific virus infections
(a) anti-insulin antibodies following chickenpox virus infection
(b) anti-pancreatic B cells following mumps virus infection
(c) anti-DNA antibodies following Epstein–Barr virus infection
(d) anti-lymphocyte antibodies following human immunodeficiency virus infection
(e) anti-heart muscle antibodies following Coxsackie B virus infection

Paper 11 Antiviral agents and prophylaxis

1. **The following agents have clinically useful antiviral activity**
(a) alpha-interferon
(b) fucidin
(c) acyclovir
(d) heparin
(e) azidothymidine

2. *The following antiviral agents and mechanisms of action are matched*
(a) *amantadine and inhibition of uncoating of virus*
(b) *acyclovir and inhibition of thymidine kinase*
(c) *ribavirin and inhibition of viral maturation*
(d) *azidothymidine and inhibition of reverse transcriptase*
(e) *ganciclovir and inhibition of viral nucleic acid synthesis*

3. **The following statements are true**
(a) oral acyclovir is the treatment of choice for herpes encephalitis
(b) intravenous acyclovir is used for the treatment of varicella-zoster infection in immunocompromised patients
(c) amantadine is useful for the treatment of influenza B virus infection
(d) aerosolised ribavirin is useful for the treatment of infection due to respiratory syncytial virus
(e) dideoxyinosine (ddt) is indicated in patients intolerant of azidothymidine

4. **Recognized unwanted effects of antiviral drugs include**
(a) bone marrow suppression with azidothymidine
(b) pancreatitis with dideoxyinosine
(c) peripheral neuropathy with acyclovir
(d) emergence of pathogenic drug-resistant strains with amantadine
(e) anaemia with ribavirin

5. **Useful in the management of drug-resistant strains of herpes simplex virus are**
(a) selective use of antiviral agents
(b) cessation of acyclovir with re-implementation a few days later
(c) replacement of acyclovir with foscarnet
(d) withdrawal of immunosuppressive therapy in herpesvirus-infected renal transplant patients
(e) monitoring of virus isolates by polymerase chain reaction

6. **The following are general principles of viral vaccine use**
(a) consent must be obtained
(b) vaccination should be postponed till after recovery from acute febrile illness
(c) alcohol used to cleanse the inoculation site should be allowed to dry before administering live vaccine
(d) the dose of the vaccine should always be checked
(e) human normal immunoglobulin should not be given at the same time and site as live vaccine

7. **Contraindications to the use of live vaccines include**
(a) immunosuppression in the patient
(b) concurrent high-dose steroid therapy
(c) pregnancy
(d) previous history of severe local reaction to the same vaccine
(e) family history of adverse reaction to vaccine

8. **The following vaccines licensed for use in the UK are live**
(a) hepatitis B
(b) measles
(c) rubella
(d) yellow fever
(e) hepatitis A

Answers

Paper 1   Introduction to viruses

INTRODUCTION

1. FFTFF

Viruses can be viewed as either very complex chemicals or the simplest life forms. Although they can reproduce, they cannot, by most criteria, be considered truly 'living'. They cannot replicate without using host cellular functions and they are unable to produce biochemical energy. They are, however, infectious. The free virus particle or virion has two or three basic structural features. At the core is a genome which may be DNA or RNA: this, in turn, may be single-stranded, double-stranded and/or segmented. The genome is enclosed within a protein coat, the capsid. The capsid is made up of a large number of protein subunits called capsomers. It takes one of two basic morphologies: cubic (usually icosahedral) or helical. Some viruses have features of both and are complex. Some viruses have a further outer layer, the envelope, which is derived from host membranes, and therefore contains lipid (Figure 1.1). This lipid component makes them susceptible to lose their infectivity by the action of detergents. A few viruses also have proteinaceous structures between the capsid and envelope: e.g. the tegument of herpesviruses. Some more complex viruses also contain virally-coded enzymes, such as the reverse transcriptase of human immunodeficiency virus, in the virion.

There are a number of virus-like agents. Viroids are naked cyclic single-stranded RNA molecules which cause disease in plants. Prions are putative infectious agents which consist of protein alone. These

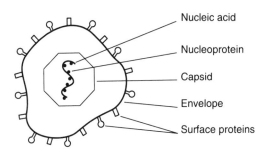

Figure 1.1 Basic structure of an enveloped virus.

are not viruses because even the simplest viruses, the so-called defective viruses that need a helper virus to replicate, possess both protein and nucleic acid.

2. TTFTF

The classification of viruses is decided by working parties of the International Committee on Taxonomy of Viruses (ICTV). Human viruses are grouped into families which have the suffix -viridae. Some families are subdivided into subfamilies, which have the suffix -virinae. There are a number of genera that constitute the families and subfamilies and these have the suffix -virus. Conventionally all these groupings are written in italics. The virus species that are members of each genus have vernacular terms and are written in Roman letters. Many schemes have been used for classifying viruses but they all, now, have as their basis structural characteristics such as the physical nature of the genome (RNA or DNA, gene sequence etc.), presence or absence of envelope, and morphology of the capsid. Currently, the same taxonomic criteria are applied to all viruses whether of plant, animal or bacterial origin. Historical anomalies, however, still exist. Basic properties of all the major virus families that include human pathogens, are shown in Table 1.1.

Table 1.1 *Major virus families that infect humans*

Family	Nucleic acid	Envelope	Capsid	Example
Adenoviridae	*dsDNA*	*No*	*Cubic*	*Adenovirus*
Arenaviridae	*ssRNA*	*Yes*	*Complex*	*Lassa*
Bunyaviridae	*ssRNA*	*Yes*	*Helical*	*Hantaan*
Caliciviridae	*ssRNA*	*No*	*Cubic*	*Norwalk virus*
Coronaviridae	*ssRNA*	*Yes*	*Helical*	*229E*
Filoviridae	*ssRNA*	*Yes*	*Helical*	*Marburg*
Flaviviridae	*ssRNA*	*Yes*	*Cubic*	*Yellow fever*
Hepadnaviridae	*dsDNA*	*No*	*Cubic*	*Hepatitis B*
Herpesviridae	*dsDNA*	*Yes*	*Cubic*	*Cytomegalovirus*
Orthomyxoviridae	*ssRNA*	*Yes*	*Helical*	*Influenza*
Papovaviridae	*dsDNA*	*No*	*Cubic*	*Papillomavirus*
Paramyxoviridae	*ssRNA*	*Yes*	*Helical*	*Respiratory syncytial*
Parvoviridae	*ssDNA*	*No*	*Cubic*	*B19*
Picornaviridae	*ssRNA*	*No*	*Cubic*	*Rhinovirus*
Poxviridae	*dsDNA*	*Yes*	*Complex*	*Molluscum contagiosum*
Reoviridae	*dsRNA*	*No*	*Cubic*	*Rotavirus*
Retroviridae	*ssRNA*	*Yes*	*Complex*	*Human immunodeficiency*
Rhabdoviridae	*ssRNA*	*Yes*	*Helical*	*Rabies*
Togaviridae	*ssRNA*	*Yes*	*Cubic*	*Rubella*

The arboviruses, derived from ar*thropod-borne viruses, share the property of being spread by arthropod vectors but include viruses from the* Arenaviridae, Bunyaviridae, Flaviviridae, Reoviridae, Rhabodoviridae *and* Togarividae.

PATHOGENESIS

3. TTFTT
There are four main routes of virus entry into the human body (Table 1.2).

Table 1.2 Routes of entry

Route	Viruses
Mucocutaneous	Human immunodeficiency viruses Hepatitis B Herpes simplex Rabies Molluscum contagiosum
Respiratory tract	Rhinoviruses Coronaviruses Adenoviruses (most) Influenza Parainfluenza Respiratory syncytial Epstein–Barr Mumps Measles Rubella Varicella-zoster BK and JC
Alimentary tract	Rotavirus Adenovirus (40 and 41) Calicivirus Enterovirus Hepatitis A Hepatitis E
Direct inoculation (bite etc.)	Hepatitis B Human immunodeficiency virus Cytomegalovirus Hepatitis C

4. TTTFT

The term 'pathogenicity' refers to the ability of an infectious agent to cause disease; virulence is a quantitative assessment of that ability. Determinants of virulence in many viruses are not well character- ized. Viral load is one important factor as the likelihood of infection in general increases with the amount of virus in the inoculum although the minimal infectious dose will vary from virus to virus and between different virus–host interactions. Strict correlation between the amount of virus and severity of clinical disease is thus not possible. Host factors determining outcome in a virus–host relationship are perhaps better known. (1) Age: adults tend to suffer more severe disease from most virus infections, e.g. pneumonia with chickenpox. (2) Genetic predisposition: there are racial differences and in some cases a specific genetic determinant has been identified. An example is sus- ceptibility to human coronavirus 229E infection which is determined by gene(s) on chromosome 15. (3) Malnutrition: children with kwa- shiorkor, for example, are susceptible to severe or fatal measles infection. (4) Immunosuppression: cell-mediated immunity and humoral responses have differing roles with different viruses. Children with severe hypogammaglobulinaemia recover normally from chickenpox and measles but are particularly susceptible to paralytic poliomyelitis. Patients with T cell deficiencies, such as those on immunosuppres- sive therapy post-transplantation, are particularly susceptible to herpesvirus infections. (5) Pre-existing antibody (either specific or cross-reactive): although this is not always protective, attenuation of illness occurs; an example would be infection with rubella virus. (6) Breastfeeding: breastfed babies appear to be less susceptible than bottle fed infants to, particularly, viruses transmitted by the faecal–oral route. (7) Psychological factors: stress and other psychological factors are known to affect the immune system. Thus it has been shown that premorbid stress increases the likelihood of infection with common cold viruses.

5. TTTTT

Both non-specific (flow of external bodily secretions, stomach acid, phagocytes, integrity of mucocutaneous surfaces) and specific (cell-mediated and humoral) factors that are active against other microbial pathogens are active against viruses. Secretory IgA is important in the prevention of mucosally acquired infection and neutralizing antibody (usually IgG1 and IgG3) is important in controlling some systemic virus infections. Interferons are unique in their antiviral activity (1.6).

6. TTFTT
Interferons are naturally-produced soluble factors that are involved in the regulation of cell growth. They are also induced in infected cells by most viruses and released extracellularly: double-stranded RNA (dsRNA) appears to be a particularly powerful inducing agent and many viruses replicate via a dsRNA intermediate. Synthesis starts at about the time of viral maturation and continues for many hours. The effect is to activate, in surrounding cells, genes that control antiviral proteins. In cells in which the virus has already replicated the antiviral effect of interferons is minimal. In general the more slowly growing a virus the higher the level of interferon produced. At least three classes of interferon are recognized. Alpha-interferon is produced mainly by polymorphonuclear leukocytes, beta-interferon by fibroblasts (although all cell types can produce this) and gamma-interferon by lymphocytes. Virus infections are best at inducing the first two classes although other infectious agents (e.g. Mycoplasma pneumoniae *and* Listeria monocytogenes*) also induce interferon, albeit at lower levels. The antiviral effects of interferon are complex but include inhibition of viral protein synthesis, prevention of egress of virus from the cell and enhancement of the immune response. These effects are not virus-specific. Exogenous interferon has similar effects to endogenous interferon and has been used therapeutically.*

7. TTTTT
The effects of viruses on cells range from almost nil to cell death: the precise effect depends on both the virus and the cell. The discernible damage is known as cytopathic effect (CPE). The most obvious effect is cell death. Viral proteins shut down host cell macromolecular synthesis and divert it to viral protein synthesis. Viruses such as polioviruses are cytocidal. Accumulation of viral proteins, which may be seen as inclusion bodies, may also be toxic and incompatible with survival of the cell. Inclusion bodies may be intracytoplasmic (poxviruses, paramyxoviruses, reoviruses, rhabdoviruses) or intranuclear (adenoviruses, herpesviruses). Cell fusion, forming syncytia, can result from the effect of viral fusion proteins. The paramyxoviruses are particularly adept at doing this, both in vivo *and in cultured cells. Other obvious cellular changes such as pyknosis (dense, shrunken nuclei) and 'cloudy' swelling of cells are caused by other viruses. Transformation of cells occurs with some DNA viruses (hepatitis B, papillomaviruses, herpesviruses, adenoviruses) and retroviruses. Integration into the host chromosome is a feature of most of these viruses. There is now convincing evidence for the causative role of a number of viruses in the genesis of cancers:*

hepatitis B and primary hepatocellular carcinoma, Epstein–Barr virus and African Burkitt's lymphoma, human T cell lymphotropic virus and adult T cell leukaemia. Steady state persistent infection results in minimal effects on the host cell. This has been shown to occur with a number of RNA viruses (arenaviruses, paramyxoviruses, retroviruses). The actual mechanism by which the virus causes disease in the host is a result of many of these effects. Also, in some virus infections, the immune system plays an important role in the pathogenesis.

8. FTFTF
A simplified version of the replication cycle of a virus is shown in Figure 1.2. Viruses enter cells by a specific interaction with a receptor protein; this is the basis of tissue tropism. If enveloped, the envelope fuses with most membranes. Once within the cell the virus uncoats to release the genome. For replication, the genome must be converted, if necessary, to positive-sense (i.e. messenger) RNA. Production of new virions may start in the cytoplasm or nucleus (or both). In general, DNA virus

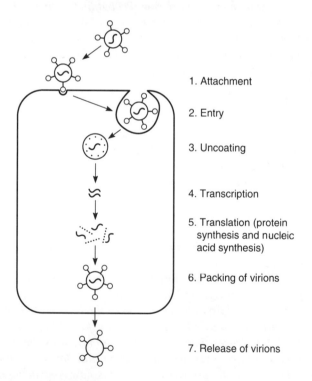

1. Attachment

2. Entry

3. Uncoating

4. Transcription

5. Translation (protein synthesis and nucleic acid synthesis)

6. Packing of virions

7. Release of virions

Figure 1.2 *Basic steps in the replication cycle of a virus.*

transcription occurs in the nucleus with translation in the cytoplasm; the exceptions are the poxviruses which replicate entirely in the cytoplasm. RNA viruses (with the exception of retroviruses) replicate in the cytoplasm. All these steps are potential targets for antiviral agents. The few drugs that have been made available for clinical use target uncoating (amantadine and derivatives), nucleic acid and protein synthesis (acyclovir, azidothymidine, ribavirin, foscarnet and related compounds) or virus release (foscarnet, amantadine).

LABORATORY DIAGNOSIS

9. TFTTT

The site and timing of sampling of specimens are possibly the most important factors for successful virus diagnosis. In general, specimens should be taken from site of symptoms, e.g. vesicles in herpes labialis, and as close to the onset of illness as possible. Additional specimens, e.g. urine for mumps virus, may also be useful. Immediate transit to the laboratory (at least within 24 hours) minimizes loss of infectivity of the virus; as does the use of an antibiotic-containing buffered viral transport medium. If delay of more than an hour is anticipated specimens are best kept at 4 °C. An acute phase serum should also be considered at this early stage. In cases where a retrospective diagnosis has to be made, a fourfold rise in specific antibody levels compared with a convalescent serum taken 10–14 days later is usually indicative of infection.

10. FFFFF

Viruses can be detected in one of four main ways: detection of virus directly, detection of viral antigens, detection of viral nucleic acid and detection of antiviral antibody. Viruses may need to be grown before they can be detected. This can be by culture in cell monolayers, eggs or animals. Egg and animal culture are becoming less popular and are reserved for specific viruses such as Coxsackie A viruses (in newborn mice). Cell monolayer culture (with allied confirmatory tests if required) is the standard by which all other more direct detection methods are compared. There are two principal types of cell used: cell strains and continuous cell lines. Cell strains are differentiated cells which still have the characteristics of their tissue of origin. They support the growth of a wide range of viruses but are limited to about 50 cycles of growth and are therefore more cumbersome to use in diagnostic laboratories because fresh cells need to be frequently prepared. Continuous cell lines are transformed cells which like other malignant cells can be considered 'immortal'. They are much more uniform than cell strains and support the growth of fewer viruses. Virus replication in cell culture can be detected by five means: (1) observation of cellular changes and death (cytopathic effect, CPE), (2) adsorption of red cells (haemadsorption), (3) interference of CPE produced by other viruses, (4) antigen detection, and (5) electron microscopic visualization of virus progeny in supernatant. Direct identification of virus is by electron microscopy; strictly this is the detection of the shadow cast by a virus as the negative stains used, such as tungsten or uranium salts, stain the area around a virus not the virus itself. The technique is widely used for the detection of diarrhoeal viruses but is limited in its use for other specimens as the lower limit of sensitivity is of the order of 10^6 organisms/ml specimen. Enhancements such as the use of antibody-coated solid phases to capture virus (solid-phase immune electron microscopy, SPIEM) improve the sensitivity.

Detection of viral antigens can be achieved by a number of antibody-dependent techniques: immunofluorescence (IF), latex agglutination (LA), haemagglutination-inhibition (HAI), neutralization, reverse-passive haemagglutination (RPH), complement fixation (CFT), enzyme-linked immunoassay (ELISA) and radioimmunoassay (RIA). Direct immunofluorescence utilizes a single fluorescein-labelled antibody to bind to specific antigens of the virus. The fluorescein label can then be seen using a fluorescent microscope. Indirect immunofluorescence uses two antibodies, one to bind to the virus and the other to bind to the first. The second antibody is labelled. Sensitivity is increased and only a single labelled antibody need be made for the detection of any virus. Immunofluorescence offers rapid diagnosis and has been particularly useful in the diagnosis of respiratory virus infections. Latex agglutination is a simple test that employs latex particles which have been coated with specific antibody so that agglutination occurs from cross-linking in the presence of antigen. It has gained acceptance for the detection of rotavirus infections. Neutralization is a well-established methodology. In common use, it depends on the inhibition of viral CPE by the prior addition of specific antiserum to a virus. As the titre of serum required can be determined, it gives an estimate of the amount of virus in a sample. It is used to confirm that the CPE seen in cell culture is due to a specific virus. ELISA and RIA (see below) are sensitive methods that can detect a few nanograms of antigen. ELISA is becoming the test of choice as it is amenable to the processing of large numbers of specimens and automation. Reverse passive haemagglutination is still used in some laboratories for the detection of hepatitis B antigen but is being superseded by ELISA.

The detection of anti viral antibody in patient serum or bodily secretions (such as urine or saliva) can be made by those techniques listed for the detection of antigen; in addition single radial haemolysis is used for rubella antibody screening. HAI is useful for those viruses, e.g. influenza, which haemagglutinate red cells; specific antibody present will prevent the phenomenon. CFT is based on the principle that in the presence of antibody and complement sensitized red cells with antigen on their surface are lysed. If this complement is adsorbed ('fixed') by antigen-antibody in test sera, an indicator system consisting of sensitized red cells, anti-red cell serum and the test serum will not result in cell lysis. CFT is used as a screening test for antibodies to a large number of antigens. Titration of test serum gives an estimate of the level of antibody present. Usually a rise in antibody level between paired sera is sought but a single high antibody titre to some agents, e.g. influenza and *Mycoplasma pneumoniae*, is highly suggestive. The test is technically demanding and has been replaced by ELISA in many laboratories. RIA and ELISA utilize the same principles. In its simplest form, antigen is bound to a solid phase so that specific antibody in a serum sample will bind to it and so indirectly to the solid phase. A labelled antihuman antibody is then added to detect the presence of the bound serum antibody. In RIA the label is a radioisotope and in ELISA an enzyme that has a chromogenic substrate that can be added. Although RIA formats are often more sensitive, ELISA tests are preferable as they do not use radioisotopes.

Detection of viral nucleic acid has the theoretical advantage that non-infectious virus as well as intact virions can be detected. Until recently the methodology has proved too cumbersome for routine diagnostic use. The advent of a technique that amplifies genes, the polymerase chain reaction (PCR), has changed this. This technique is very sensitive and can potentially detect a single virus in a clinical specimen. Commercially-available diagnostic kits are being introduced at the time of writing of this book.

CONTROL OF INFECTION

11. TTTTF
Although there are few hard data to support it, it is generally assumed that standard methods of sterilization (Table 1.3) for bacteria are effective against viruses. On the other hand, most disinfectants used in clinical practice are unreliable in their activity against viruses, particularly non-enveloped viruses. Enveloped viruses in general are more susceptible because of the lipid nature of the envelope that

can be solubilized by detergents. Phenolics (e.g. 'Hycolin'), quaternary ammonium compounds (e.g. cetrimide), chlorhexidine and hexachlorophane have no or little activity against viruses. Seventy per cent alcohol is useful against most enveloped viruses and has been shown to be useful in the prevention of transmission of rotaviruses (but not other enteric viruses). More reliable agents are 2% glutaraldehyde, peroxygen compounds (e.g. 'Virkon'), formaldehyde and hypochlorite. The last of these is the most commonly used: a solution of 10 000 parts per million (ppm) active chlorine (a 10% solution of strong domestic bleach) is useful for heavily contaminated surfaces and 1000 ppm for less obviously contaminated surfaces. As the use of these agents is less effective in the presence of organic material, prior washing is a prerequisite. Glutaraldehyde (2%) for 30–60 minutes is useful for disinfecting metal instruments such as endoscopes and if used for 12 hours is sterilizing. Handwashing is an integral part of reducing viral contamination and transmission.

Table 1.3 Sterilization methods for viruses

Method	Example of operating conditions	Applications
Laboratory autoclave	121°C for 15 minutes	Glassware, solutions, plastic laboratory discard
Steam with formalin	73°C for 3 hours	Heat-sensitive equipment
Ethylene oxide	60°C, 100% ethylene oxide for 12 hours	Heat-sensitive equipment
Glutaraldehyde (2%)	12 hours	Metal instruments

12. TFFTF

Patients with infection due to viruses are isolated for one (or both) of two reasons: (1) the viruses are highly infectious and are a potential risk of serious infection in some patients; or (2) they cause serious infection in the population generally. Measles and chickenpox are examples of infections in the first group. The latter group are so-called category III and IV pathogens (Table 1.4): these categories are used in laboratories and apply to agents that pose a threat of serious disease. Specimens from patients in category IV should not be sent to laboratories without prior discussion. Most other viruses are in category II. The principles of infection control of viruses include: (1) education regarding the risks and transmission characteristics of viral pathogens, (2) barrier nursing and precautions regarding the handling of potentially infected material (Table 1.5 summarizes precautions), (3) vaccination of high-risk staff, (4) the use of aseptic technique, (5) regular cleaning and disinfection of potentially contaminated areas, (6) appropriate design of hospitals, e.g. air-conditioning that does not duct from room to room, (7) the design of outbreak management policies that can be rapidly implemented, (8) separation of immunocompromised patients from infectious risk, and (9) training of staff in hygienic practices.

Table 1.4 Dangerous viral pathogens

Biosafety category	Virus
III[a]	Herpesvirus B
	Rabies
	Vesicular stomatitis virus
	Louping ill
	Lymphocytic choriomeningitis
	Chikungunya
	Murray Valley encephalitis
	Japanese B encephalitis
	Hantaan
	Powassan
	Yellow fever
	Rift valley fever
	Venezualan encephalitis
IV	Marburg
	Ebola
	Junin
	Lassa
	Machupo
	Crimean–Congo haemorrhagic
	Tick-borne encephalitis complex

[a] Does not include some vertebrate viruses which are rarely associated with human disease. Under certain circumstances viruses such as hepatitis B and HIV will also be category III pathogens

13. TTFFT
There are regional differences in the diseases that have to be reported by law (Table 1.6). HIV is not yet a notifiable disease although laboratory diagnoses are routinely reported.

Table 1.5 Centers for Disease Control (CDC) (USA) category specific isolation standards

Category	Single room	Gown	Gloves	Masks	Hand-washing	Examples
Strict	Yes	Yes	Yes	Yes	Yes	Lassa
Respiratory	Yes	No	No	Close contact only	Yes	Measles
Contact	Yes	If soiling likely	Yes	Close contact only	Yes	Chickenpox
Enteric	Possibly	If soiling likely	If in contact with infected material	No	Yes	Norwalk
Drainage/secretion	No	If soiling likely	If in contact with infected material	No	Yes	Congenital rubella
Blood/body fluid	Possibly	If soiling likely	If in contact with infected material	No	Yes	HIV, hepatitis B

Table 1.6 Notifiable virus infections in the UK

Acute encephalitis (not Scotland)
Acute meningitis (Northern Ireland only)
Acute poliomyelitis
Chickenpox (not England and Wales)
Food poisoning
Gastroenteritis (Northern Ireland only)
Lassa fever (separate category in England and Wales only)
Measles
Mumps
Rabies
Rubella
Smallpox
Viral haemorrhagic fever
Viral hepatitis
Yellow fever (not Scotland)

14. TTTTT

Effective management of occupational exposure in healthcare workers requires rapid reporting (within 24 hours) of incidents to responsible staff. Wounds should be cleaned initially. Assessment of exposure (type of exposure, whether there is skin puncture, site of exposure, volume of blood contamination and source of exposure) and immune status of the patient should be made. If the infectivity status of the donor is unknown then testing for HBsAg, HIV and hepatitis C antibody should be considered. Concomitant use of hepatitis B immunoglobulin (within 7 days) and hepatitis B vaccine should also be considered. The use of prophylactic azidothymidine is far more controversial but is considered in some centres if it can be given within a few hours of high-risk exposure. Follow-up serology for HIV, hepatitis B and hepatitis C may be required (CDC recommend 6 weeks, 3 months and 6 months). Prevention of transmission of blood-borne viruses depends on general measures such as good hygiene practices, handwashing, the covering of cuts and exposed skin lesions and training of staff. Double-gloving is recommended for invasive procedures. The use of gowns, face masks and all-body suits may be merited under conditions of exposure to large volumes of infected blood. Hepatitis B vaccination of all staff handling patients and blood/blood products should be routine.

15. TFFFF

Needlestick injuries are the most likely scenario for the transmission of blood-borne viruses from infected patient to HCW. The risk of transmission of HIV has been calculated on epidemiological grounds to be 0.31% compared with 7–68% for heterosexual intercourse. That of hepatitis B from a HBeAg-positive contaminated needlestick is much higher at 20–30% (comparable to heterosexual transmission). There is less data for hepatitis C but in one study it was 2.7%. Recent reports of transmission of HIV from dental surgeons to patients have highlighted the risks of transmission of blood-borne viruses from infected HCW to patient. CDC (USA) have estimated the risk of transmission of HIV to be 1 in 2.4–24 million and of hepatitis B at 0.06%.

Paper 2 Viruses and the respiratory tract

INTRODUCTION

1. FTFFT

Respiratory tract infections vie with gastrointestinal infections as the major cause of mortality worldwide. Non-bacterial agents are responsible for over 90% of identifiable upper respiratory tract infections and over 30% of identifiable lower respiratory tract infections although this latter figure is likely to be an underestimate as a substantial proportion are usually not identified. The commonest syndrome is the common cold. There are a number of agents associated with this illness: rhinoviruses, coronaviruses, adenoviruses, parainfluenza viruses, respiratory syncytial virus, influenza viruses, enteroviruses, varicella-zoster virus, herpes simplex virus, Epstein–Barr virus, measles virus, *Mycoplasma pneumoniae* and group A streptococci. Rhinoviruses (30–50%) and coronaviruses (15–35%) are responsible for the majority of cases. Respiratory tract infections are an even more important cause of both morbidity and mortality in the developing world. On a worldwide basis, 98% of all deaths in 1–4 year olds from respiratory tract infections occur in countries ʾwith an infant mortality greater than 100 per 1000 population. This is from a greater severity of disease rather than greater incidence; infants in both Michigan (USA) and India have six episodes of respiratory infection per year. Socioeconomic and nutritional factors appear to be the most important. Transmission of respiratory viruses may be by either aerosol or fomites. The relative contribution of each is likely to be different for different viruses.

2. TTFTT

There are a large number of viral respiratory tract pathogens. In general any of these viruses can infect any part of the respiratory tract but specific viruses have a predilection for certain anatomical areas (Table 2.1). Parainfluenza viruses are the commonest agents causing 'croup' or laryngotracheobronchitis and respiratory syncytial virus that of bronchiolitis. Toroviruses are newly recognized viruses that have been shown to be associated with diarrhoeal disease in young farm animals such as calves. They are so-called because they have the appearance of a torus when viewed with an electron microscope. They have not been associated with human disease. There is radiological evidence of pneumonia in 25-50% of children with measles. The precise aetiology has not been determined although some cases are due to the virus itself. The proportion with clinical illness is far less. Adenoviruses cause infections throughout the respiratory tract, including pharyngoconjunctival fever.

Table 2.1 Viral respiratory pathogens

Disease	Common causes	Less common causes
Rhinitis	Rhinoviruses	Respiratory syncytial virus (RSV)
	Coronaviruses	Parainfluenza viruses
		Influenza viruses
		Adenoviruses
		Enteroviruses
Pharyngitis	Parainfluenza viruses	Rhinoviruses
	Influenza viruses	Adenoviruses
	Herpes simplex	RSV
	Epstein–Barr virus	Cytomegalovirus
	Coxsackie A	
Laryngotracheobronchitis	Parainfluenza viruses (serotypes 3 more than 1, 2)	RSV
	Influenza A	Influenza B
		Adenoviruses
		Rhinoviruses
		Enteroviruses (50% unidentified)
Bronchiolitis	RSV (45-75%)	Influenza A
	Parainfluenza viruses (14-32%)	Adenoviruses
		Rhinoviruses
		Enteroviruses
Pneumonia	RSV	Adenoviruses serotypes 3, 4, 7
	Parainfluenza viruses	Measles
	Influenza viruses	Varicella
	Cytomegalovirus	

COMMON COLDS

3. TFFTF

Common colds occur worldwide. All populations and age groups are susceptible although symptomatic illness becomes less frequent with age. In the UK and USA studies have shown that on average every individual will have one cold per year. In the winter, colds caused by coronaviruses predominate whereas the peak incidence of rhinovirus colds occur in the spring and autumn. The two viruses have different incubation periods: 24–72 hours with rhinovirus colds and 12–24 hours longer with coronavirus colds. More than one serotype of each virus circulates in any particular year. Transmission of rhinoviruses may be either aerosol or fomites; the evidence for fomite transmission of coronaviruses is not available. Kissing, talking and singing are somewhat less efficient than sneezing at transmitting virus. This may be a reflection of the particle size and the lower viral load in salivary secretions. Transmission of virus may occur from asymptomatic individuals as 20% have been shown to excrete virus for 2 weeks after they have recovered from illness. Volunteer studies have shown that reinfections can be induced to the same rhinovirus serotype although the importance of this in natural infection is not established.

4. FTFFT
The common cold syndrome is readily recognized by profuse nasal discharge, sneezing and sore throat. These last for about a week with maximal symptoms in the first 2–3 days. Some systemic features such as headache occur in the majority but others such as diarrhoea, myalgia and cervical lymphadenopathy are less common. Fever occurs in less than 1% of rhinovirus colds which is a useful distinguishing feature from influenza. Complications include sinusitis and otitis media. Pneumonia, either viral or due to secondary bacterial infection, is an unusual complication. Of great interest has been the role of common cold viruses in inducing exacerbations of illness in asthmatics and chronic bronchitis; recent studies suggest that these viruses are responsible for the overwhelming majority of wheezy attacks in children. There is a school of thought that believes that infections due to respiratory viruses in the first year of life cause the damage that subsequently results in asthma.

5. FFTFT
The aim of current management of common colds is to provide symptomatic relief. Apart from adequate hydration and stopping smoking, over the counter medicines are commonly used. Agents used in over the counter medicines include antihistamines, sympathomimetics (decongestants), antitussives, analgesics, caffeine, anticholinergic compounds and alcohol. Vitamin C has also been advocated but clinical trials have not consistently supported the benefit of even high-dose vitamin C. Zinc lozenges have theoretical activity against rhinovirus colds and when used at the onset of a cold have been shown to reduce the severity and duration of cold symptoms. Attempts at specific

treatment started with interferon. A spray of alpha-interferon given intranasally as a prophylactic agent does appear to reduce the incidence of colds but the side-effect rate of 10% and the cost are prohibitive. Specific anti-rhinoviral agents, such as enviroxime, dichloroflavan and chalcones, have been shown, despite *in vitro* activity, to be suppressive at best when used in human volunteers. The use of hot humid air to raise the internal temperature of the nose has been shown to give immediate symptomatic relief but the theoretical action of suppressing virus growth is poorly substantiated.

PHARYNGITIS

6. FTTTF
Streptococcus pyogenes is the commonest single identifiable cause of acute pharyngitis (15–30% of all cases). Rhinoviruses (20%), coronaviruses (5%), adenoviruses (5%), herpes simplex (2%), parainfluenza (2%) and influenza A (2%) are also commonly found. All other identifiable causes (coxsackie A, EBV, CMV, HIV and non-viral causes) are each thought to be responsible for less than 1% of cases. A significant minority (up to 40%) do not have a diagnosable cause. The specific diagnosis depends usually on culture of throat swabs that have been transported in viral transport medium.

LARYNGITIS

7. TFTTT
Viruses are responsible for the majority of cases of acute laryngitis. Influenza, rhinoviruses and adenovirus appear to be the most frequent. Parainfluenza, coxsackie A21 and coronaviruses are less commonly implicated.

RHINOVIRUS

8. TFTTT
Rhinoviruses are members of the **Picornaviridae**. *Like the other members of this genus, they possess non-enveloped capsids with icosahedral symmetry of about 28 nm diameter. The nucleocapsid consists of four structural proteins (VP1–4) surrounding a single strand of positive sense RNA. They can be distinguished from the enteroviruses by their*

acid lability (this property makes them susceptible to stomach acid when swallowed). There are more than 110 serotypes recognized by specific neutralizing antibodies. Sequencing of the genomes has confirmed variability in those regions which are translated into antigens that induce neutralizing antibody (suggesting a single vaccine is unlikely) but there is significant conservation in other regions (useful for gene diagnosis). These serotypes can be grouped into two major types in accordance with host receptor specificity. Most rhinoviruses (90%) will bind to the host protein intracellular adhesion molecule 1 (ICAM-1) or 'major' receptor but others utilize another 'minor' receptor. This is not dissimilar to an older classification into M and H types: H types (broadly equivalent to the 'major' group) only replicate in cells of human origin, M types in both human and monkey cells. The single strand of RNA codes for a single polyprotein that is then cleaved to produce the capsid proteins. It is thought that zinc, which has been used as treatment, may inhibit this post-translational cleavage step.

CORONAVIRUS

9. TTFTF

Coronaviruses are enveloped viruses of 80–120 nm in diameter. They have a characteristic morphology with a 'crown' of spikes projecting from the virion surface. The family **Coronaviridae** *is comprised of viruses that infect humans, birds and mammals; recently a related group of viruses, the toroviruses, have been included in this family. They possess a single strand of RNA of positive polarity, at over 27 kb the longest viral RNA genome recognized so far. This RNA, via an intermediate negative sense copy, is transcribed into six 'nested' subgenomic size mRNAs which are coterminous at the 3' end. The major structural proteins produced are a surface peplomer (S), a membrane or matrix protein (M) which is inserted into the envelope and a nucleocapsid protein (N) intertwined with the RNA. Some coronaviruses have a second, smaller, surface projection formed from a haemagglutinin protein. There are at least two major human serotypes with the prototype strains being 229E and OC43. Apart from being responsible for 15–35% of all common colds, coronaviruses have been associated with lower respiratory tract infection. Less certain is their role in causing diarrhoeal disease. The viruses have also been associated with thyroiditis, hepatitis and multiple sclerosis but there is little evidence to support an aetiological role. Over 70% of individuals in temperate climates will have serum antibody to both coronavirus strains by the age of 30 years but reinfections* are still common. Immunity wanes over a period of 1–4 years after infection. Currently there is not a good animal model for studying human coronavirus infections.

PARAINFLUENZA VIRUS

10. FTTTF

Parainfluenza viruses are members of the **Paramyxoviridae**. These are spherical enveloped viruses of 125–150 nm in diameter. They possess a single-stranded RNA genome of negative polarity. The viral capsid contains proteins inserted through the envelope which have haemagglutinin, neuraminidase and fusion properties within the same structure. There are four serotypes recognized, termed 1–4; type 4 is also subtyped into 4a and 4b. Parainfluenza type 3 infections are experienced early in life: 50% of children are seropositive by the age of 1 year. Parainfluenza types 1 and 2 have a slightly later peak but the majority of infections still occur in pre-school children. The peak time for parainfluenza virus infections in temperate climates is the winter. Co-circulation of types occurs throughout the year. Transmission of parainfluenza viruses is thought to be mainly by droplets and there does not appear to be an animal reservoir. Laboratory diagnosis of infection can be made by culture of the virus in primate cells or by a rise in antibody level although this latter method is complicated by serological cross-relativity between human types and animal parainfluenza viruses. Direct immunofluorescence of respiratory secretions enables the most rapid diagnosis. Live attenuated vaccines have shown promise in primate studies but extensive data on their use in humans are not yet available. Amantadine and its derivatives do not have in vitro activity against parainfluenza viruses. Ribavirin has in vitro activity but its role in clinical management is yet to be defined.

11. TFTTF

Coryzal symptoms occur in both adults and children after an incubation period of 2 days. In children these may develop into laryngotracheobronchitis which is the predominant parainfluenza virus-related illness resulting in hospitalization. The same illness can be caused by influenza viruses, respiratory syncytial virus and *Mycoplasma pneumoniae*. The illness comprises fever, coryza, sore throat, hoarseness and increased breathing difficulty. An X-ray may show 'the steeple sign' of subglottic narrowing. The differential diagnosis is mainly from bacterial tracheitis caused by *Staphylococcus aureus* which may have an identical clinical picture. Pneumonia occurs less frequently in both adults and children but at particular risk are those with severe combined immunodeficiency. Parotitis can also occur. A reported association with Paget's disease of bone has not been substantiated by sensitive gene detection methods. Reinfection with the same serotype does occur but is uncommon in comparison with other respiratory viruses. Shedding of virus occurs from 8 to 11 days after infection, but rarely longer.

RESPIRATORY SYNCYTIAL VIRUS

12. TFTFT

*Respiratory syncytial virus (RSV) is an atypical member of the **Paramyxoviridae**. Differences from the other members of the virus family place it in a separate genus,* Pneumovirus. *It possesses a single strand of negative-sense RNA which codes for surface proteins with fusion (F) and attachment (G) properties; the virus lacks haemagglutinin and neuraminidase activity. It is not a hardy virus and may not remain infectious after freezing. There are two serogroups recognized by monoclonal antibody typing based on differences in both the F and G proteins. These have been termed A and B. Strains from both subgroups co-circulate with one subgroup predominant in any specific year. There is some evidence to suggest that subgroup A infections are more severe. Transmission is thought to be by direct inoculation of the nose with aerosols playing a minor role. Diagnosis of infection has become more common since the advent of specific antiviral therapy with ribavirin. Direct immunofluorescence of respiratory secretions is usually attempted with culture in cell monolayers (HEp-2, monkey kidney) for confirmation. Other antigen detection systems based on ELISA, RIA and SRH are less frequently used. Serology is useful for epidemiological studies. The antiviral, ribavirin, has in* vitro *activity against RSV. It is delivered by aerosol and has been shown to decrease the severity of illness. There is little toxicity with its use in this form. Use of the drug is particularly recommended for infection in three classes of patients: (1) children with chronic cardiovascular or pulmonary disease, prematurity and those with immunodeficiency; these patients are at risk of severe disease; (2) children with severe lower respiratory tract disease; and (3) children less than 6 weeks of age or with congenital anomalies. A number of vaccines (both live and killed) have been tried in the past without success. Indeed, in one early study subsequent infection with RSV led to more severe lower respiratory tract disease in those with prior vaccination than those without. One explanation for this* *may be the important role that the immune response has in the pathogenesis of lower respiratory tract disease.*

13. FTFFT

RSV epidemics occur annually in temperate climates. They show sharp peaks of about 3 months duration starting December or January. Despite the presence of maternal antibody, the peak incidence of bronchiolitis is at about 2 months of age and by the age of 2 years 75% of children have serological evidence of having been exposed to RSV. Nursery schools and family units are the common settings for transmission with high penetrance of illness in susceptible children. Bronchiolitis is the commonest severe illness associated with RSV although other organisms (parainfluenza viruses, adenoviruses, influenza viruses and *Mycoplasma pneumoniae*) may also cause bronchiolitis. The illness tends to be preceded by a few days of upper respiratory tract symptoms with resolution of the clinical signs and symptoms in less than a week. Lung function abnormalities can, however, be detected for months or years. Almost half of the children will have further bouts of wheezing, making differentiation from asthma difficult. Pneumonia is less common but can occur in up to 40% of children hospitalized with bronchiolitis. Croup and otitis media are also reported complications. Adults tend to have pre-existing neutralizing antibody but still suffer infection although this tends to be restricted to common colds.

ADENOVIRUSES

14. FTTFT

Adenoviruses (family **Adenoviridae***) are non-enveloped viruses of approximately 80 nm diameter with a characteristic icosahedral symmetry. Within the capsid is a genome of double-stranded DNA. There are at least ten proteins associated with the capsid which form hexons at the face of the icosahedron and pentons at the vertices. From the pentons projects an attachment protein, the fibre. The viruses are relatively hardy, remaining infectious for several weeks at 4°C and after exposure to lipid solvents. Heating to 56°C results in loss of infectivity within 5 minutes. Human adenoviruses can be classified into at least 47 serotypes in six subgenera (A–F). Types 43–47 have only been found to date in patients with AIDS. Alternative typing schemes based on DNA homology have concordance with the serological methods. The viruses are readily propagated in human continuous cell lines such as HeLa or HEp-2 cells; alternatively primary cultures such as HEK cells* *can be used. This is the standard means of detection in respiratory secretions but 2–20 days elapse before CPE is detectable. More rapid diagnosis is achieved by direct immunofluorescence or ELISA although both lack sensitivity when compared with culture. Supportive information is provided by serology (CFT or ELISA). There is no specific therapy for adenovirus infections; neither idoxuridine nor adenine arabinoside have proved to be therapeutically useful in eye infections. Vaccines have been produced against serotypes 3, 4, 7 and 21. In the USA, military recruits are immunized against types 4 and 7, the vaccine induces neutralizing antibody in over 75%.*

15. TTTFT

Adenoviruses have been associated with a wide spectrum of illness (Table 2.2). Adenovirus types 1, 2 and 5 are recognized as being endemic in North America and Europe. Most infections caused by these serotypes are asymptomatic but they still result in 5% of all paediatric respiratory disease in these areas. The incubation period of endemic disease is 5–10 days with the clinical illness manifest as fever (over 80%), pharyngitis, tonsillitis and cough. Coryza, diarrhoea and vomiting, meningism and pneumonia occur less frequently. In patients with pneumonia, hilar lymphadenopathy appears to be a common chest X-ray feature. Acute respiratory disease is the name given to a syndrome characterized by fever, pharyngitis, cervical lymphadenopathy, cough and malaise. The illness occurs in epidemic form particularly in military recruits. In this latter group the peak incidence is within 3 weeks of starting military training with 10% developing pneumonia and requiring hospitalization. Resolution of illness is in 2–3 weeks. Pharyngoconjunctival fever is characterized by fever, conjunctivitis and mild pharyngitis in association with prior swimming activity in swimming pools with inadequate chlorination. The illness lasts 7–8 days, usually without permanent eye damage. Epidemic keratoconjunctivitis (EKC) is characterized by follicular conjunctivitis with pain, photophobia and lacrimation. Progression may occur to corneal erosions and systemic features such as fever and malaise. It affects predominantly males between the ages of 20 and 40 years and because of an association with shipyard workers it has been known as 'shipyard eye'. Transmission is by direct inoculation. The illness subsides in 4–6 weeks but may leave subepithelial corneal opacities and scarring. Skin infections are uncommon and are morbilliform or rubelliform.

Table 2.2 Adenovirus serotypes associated with disease

Disease	Serotypes
Acute pharyngitis	**1** 2 3 **5** 6 7
Pharyngoconjunctival fever	1 2 **3** 4 6 **7** 14
Epidemic keratoconjunctivitis	**8** 11 **19 37**
Follicular conjunctivitis	3 4 11
Acute respiratory disease	3 **4 7** 11 14 21
Pertussis-like syndrome	**5**
Pneumonia	1 2 **3 4 7** 21
Gastroenteritis	9 12 18 25 26 27 28 **40 41** 42
Acute haemorrhagic cystitis	1 4 7 **11 21**
Intussusception	1 2 5
Cervicitis/urethritis	**37**
Immunocompromised (includes AIDS)	5 32 34 35 36 43 44 45 46 47
Disseminated	4 5 7 **34 35**
Hepatitis	3 5 7
Skin infections	2 4 7 21
Acute febrile polyarthritis	7

The commoner serotypes reported are in bold

INFLUENZA VIRUS

16. FTFTF
Influenza viruses are members of the **Orthomyxoviridae***. There are three influenza viruses recognized (A, B and C) with C being less closely related. They are all enveloped viruses of approximately 80–120 nm in diameter. The virions may be spherical, elongated or filamentous with glycosylated protein peplomers on the surface; these are of two types in influenza A and B, a neuraminidase (N) and haemagglutinin (H) protein. Influenza C has both of these properties resident on a single protein. All three viruses have segmented RNA genomes of negative polarity: influenza A and B have eight segments, influenza C seven. A high degree of homology exists between the corresponding genes of influenza A and B but not C. Each RNA codes for one or two unique polypeptides. Replication is in the cytoplasm.*

17. FTTFF
An influenza or influenza-like illness was described by Hippocrates in the fifth century BC although the term was not used until 1358 by the Italians. Records show that there have been epidemics since at least 1510 and pandemics since 1580. The causative viruses were not however

discovered until 1933 (influenza A), 1940 (influenza B) and 1950 (influenza C). Influenza remains a major disease mainly because of the continual antigenic variation that influenza A undergoes. The most important changes occur in the surface glycoproteins of the virus (H and N proteins). The H protein is the more important as it induces neutralizing antibody whereas antibodies produced against N interfere with the systemic spread of the virus. Gradual antigenic change, due predominantly to a small number of nucleotide changes in the genes, results in 'antigenic drift'. This causes the annual 'epidemics' of illness. Major antigenic changes due to genetic reassortment between different strains result in 'pandemics'. Monitoring of the prevalent strains of influenza A by antigenic typing of the H and N proteins is used to indicate the vaccine strains required in any particular year. The prevalent strain is usually designated by its antigenic structure and reputed source, e.g. influenza A H3N2 (Hong Kong). There are 13 H and 9 N subtypes recognized. Influenza B and C undergo antigenic drift but not shift. There are a few theories of the genetic origin of new strains of influenza A. One popular hypothesis is that genes are swapped between human and animal strains in those animals that act as reservoirs of human virus, e.g. ducks and pigs. These animals do not appear to get an identical illness to that of humans, with the notable exception of ferrets. Influenza B and C probably infect humans only. Influenza affects all ages but the highest attack rates occur in pre-school children; attack rates in epidemics have been between 35 and 62% in published studies. The rate of infection and illness is less in the elderly but there is significant associated mortality in those over 65 years of age and those over 45 years with diabetes, chronic heart or chronic lung disease.

18. TTFFT

Epidemic influenza tends to occur during the cold months, i.e. late autumn to early spring in the northern hemisphere. Influenza A epidemics have a 2–3 year cycle while influenza B epidemics are every 4–6 years. Pandemics are caused by influenza A only. Transmission of the virus is by person-to-person spread with the peak of an epidemic occurring within 2–3 weeks of onset. The route of transmission is probably via aerosols although fomite transmission may play a role: the virus can remain infectious for up to 24 hours on non-porous surfaces. The incubation period is usually 18–72 hours although it may be as long as 4 days. The onset of illness is typically abrupt with predominant systemic symptoms in the early phase. Table 2.3 shows the main symptoms encountered. In general, influenza C causes a milder illness than either influenza A or B which are indistinguishable. Complications of influenza infection include co- or super-infection with other agents (*Mycoplasma pneumoniae, Legionella, Streptococcus pneumoniae, Staphylococcus aureus, Haemophilus influenzae* and *Neisseria meningitidis*) which can result in either pneumonia or meningitis. Other recognized complications include myocarditis, pericarditis, meningoencephalitis, myositis and acute myoglobinuric renal failure. Guillain–Barré syndrome has been associated with the swine flu vaccine but not those human vaccines in current use. Reye's syndrome has been associated with influenzal illness in children and concurrent salicylate usage. Mortality occurs during epidemics and pandemics in both children and the elderly.

Table 2.3 Prevalence of symptoms and signs of influenza in children and adults

Clinical feature	Adults (%)	Children (%)
Sudden onset	46	66
Fever (> 37.7°C)	87	89
Headache	72	81
Malaise	67	68
Cough	90	86
Nasal discharge	82	67
Sore throat	62	62
Conjunctivitis	56	61
Sputum production	41	19
Abdominal pain	0	31
Vomiting	7	26
Nausea	4	23
Diarrhoea	0	2
Cervical lymphadenopathy	8	38
Myalgia	62	33

19. TTFFF

The diagnosis of infection with influenza viruses can be made by growing virus in cell monolayers or hens' eggs. Cell lines that have been shown to support the growth of influenza A and B include primary monkey kidney cells and green monkey kidney cells. Influenza C grows best on a continuous monkey kidney cell line, LLC-MK2. Egg culture is rarely routinely attempted now, with the possible exception of vaccine strains. Growth in cell culture may take several days and cytopathic effects are difficult to discern. Haemadsorption of infected monolayers enhances the speed and sensitivity. More rapid diagnosis still can be made by direct immunofluorescence of respiratory secretions. Whatever the test, specimens are best taken in the first two days of illness. Serum antibody detection (HAI, SRH, CFT, ELISA) has been used in epidemiological surveys. Detection of antibody does not predict immunity to infection as reinfections are common although higher levels of antibody reduce the likelihood of infection. It is likely that local specific IgA and cell-mediated immune mechanisms are more important in protection against disease. Amantadine, and its derivative rimantidine, when used prophylactically in influenza A outbreaks have been shown to provide a protection rate of up to 75%. Rimantidine has fewer side-effects and may become accepted as the agent of choice. Both drugs are given orally as a routine although inhalational preparations are now available. The use of these agents therapeutically is less clear particularly as drug resistance is known to occur. Other agents such as inosoprine and ribavirin (which is also active *in vitro* against influenza B) have also been tried. Influenza vaccines have now been available for over 50 years. Current vaccines are grown in embryonated hens' eggs, inactivated with formalin and then purified. Formulations are generally trivalent with two prevalent strains of influenza A and one of influenza B. Efficacy is 60–80% after a single injection although the elderly have a poorer response rate. Protection lasts for about a year. The vaccines are well tolerated although local reactions are common. They are recommended to be given to high-risk populations: residents of nursing homes (particularly the elderly); those with chronic respiratory, heart, renal and lung diseases; patients with diabetes mellitus and other endocrine disorders; and the immunosuppressed. In an outbreak, the immune response to vaccine may take 2 weeks to develop and interim antiviral prophylaxis should be considered.

OTHER VIRUSES

20. TTTFT

Measles and varicella-zoster virus can cause pneumonia in the immuno-competent and immunocompromised; primary infection in adults is more likely to lead to this than in children. Other herpes viruses, herpes simplex and cytomegalovirus, rarely cause pneumonia in the overtly immuno-competent patient but are increasingly seen in patients with AIDS and those on immunosuppressive therapy after transplantation. Pneumonia in these patients is also likely to be life-threatening whereas it is a relatively trivial illness in the immunocompetent. Inoue–Melnick virus is a putative herpesvirus that has been associated with subacute myelo-opticoneuropathy, a paralysing condition reported in Japan and the USA in the 1970s.

Paper 3 Viruses and the neurological system

INTRODUCTION

1. TFTTT

Viruses are associated with a great number of neurological disorders, both obviously infectious and others (Table 3.1). The commonest disorders are meningitis and encephalitis in which enteroviruses and herpes simplex, respectively, are the primary aetiological agents. There are also agents that have been incorrectly termed 'slow viruses' that are associated with degenerative disorders such as Creutzfeld–Jakob disease. Rubella virus causes a very rare disease known as progressive rubella panencephalitis which clinically and pathologically is indistinguishable from that caused by measles virus, SSPE.

Table 3.1 Viruses and the neurological system

Disorder	Commonly associated viruses	Less commonly associated viruses
Meningitis	Enteroviruses Mumps	Herpes simplex Lymphocytic choriomeningitis Cytomegalovirus Epstein–Barr Varicella-zoster Some arboviruses (Oropouche, Toscana, Thogoto, Lipovnik, Rio Bravo)
Encephalitis	Herpes simplex Some arboviruses	Arenaviruses Bunyaviruses Rabies Enteroviruses Adenoviruses Varicella-zoster Epstein–Barr Cytomegalovirus Human immunodeficiency Measles
Post-infectious encephalomyelitis	Measles Influenza	Varicella Rubella Vaccinia Rabies vaccine

Table 3.1 *cont.*

Disorder	Commonly associated viruses	Less commonly associated viruses
Dementia	Human immunodeficiency	
Progressive multifocal leuco-encephalopathy	Polyomavirus JC	
Subacute sclerosing panencephalitis	Measles	Rubella
Paralysis	Polioviruses	Enteroviruses 70, 71 Coxsackie A7
Tropical spastic paraparesis	Human T cell leukaemia virus-1	
Guillain–Barre syndrome	Epstein–Barr Cytomegalovirus	Adenoviruses Enteroviruses Influenza A Parainfluenza-3 Swine flu vaccine
Reye's syndrome	Influenza Varicella	
Idiopathic facial palsy	Herpes simplex Varicella-zoster Mumps	Rubella Human immunodeficiency virus

3.2 FFFFF

The epidemiology of neurological infections due to viruses reflects the epidemiology of the principal viruses. Thus viral meningitis is commonest in the summer months, reflecting the predominance of enteroviruses. LCM is a member of the *Arenaviridae* and has a rodent host. Secondary transmission can occur to humans in rodent-infested areas or by laboratory-associated accidents. It is an uncommon cause of meningitis in humans and although there has been a slight winter peak, infection occurs at all times of the year. Most of the viruses that commonly cause encephalitis are found worldwide but the arthropod-borne viral encephalitides are endemic to specific regions; this reflects the epidemiology of the vector and natural host (Table 3.2). In epidemic years up to 50% of all viral encephalitides may be due to these arboviruses in endemic areas. Transmission of most non-arthropod borne viruses is by human-to-human contact but the arboviruses and rabies are zoonoses and person-to-person transmission is uncommon or unknown.

Table 3.2 Arboviral encephalitides

Virus	Family	Vector	Reservoir	Endemic areas	Mortality rate (%)
Eastern Equine Encephalitis	*Togaviridae*	Mosquito	Birds	Eastern USA, Canada, C and S America, Caribbean	50–70
Western Equine Encephalitis	*Togaviridae*	Mosquito	Birds	USA, Canada Argentina	2–3
Venezuelan Equine Encephalitis	*Togaviridae*	Mosquito	Horses, small mammals	C and S America southwestern USA	0–1
St Louis Encephalitis	*Flaviviridae*	Mosquito	Birds	USA, Canada, Caribbean, Brazil	5–20
Powassan	*Flaviviridae*	Tick	Birds, small mammals	Canada, USA former Soviet Union	Not known (too few cases)
California group	*Bunyaviridae*	Mosquito	Rodents	N and C America	2
Colorado tick fever	*Reoviridae*	Tick	Rodents	Western USA	Rare
Japanese B encephalitis	*Flaviviridae*	Mosquito	Small mammals, birds, reptiles	SE Asia, China, India	20–50
Murray Valley	*Flaviviridae*	Mosquito	Small mammals, birds	Australasia	20–60
Rocio	*Flaviviridae*	Mosquito	Mice, birds	Brazil	10–15
Tick-borne encephalitis group	*Flaviviridae*	Mosquito	Small mammals, rodents	Far East, former Soviet Union, C and N Europe	5–30
Louping ill	*Flaviviridae*	Tick	Sheep, deer	UK, Western Europe	Uncommon
Semliki Forest	*Togaviridae*	Mosquito		Africa	Not known (too few cases)
Kyasanur Forest	*Flaviviridae*	Tick	Rodents, monkeys	India	1–10
Kunjin	*Flaviviridae*	Mosquito	Rodents	India	Uncommon
West Nile	*Flaviviridae*	Mosquito	Birds	Africa, India, Middle East, Europe	Uncommon
Rift Valley Fever	*Bunyaviridae*	Mosquito	Rodents	Africa	Uncommon
Vesicular stomatitis	*Rhabdoviridae*	Phlebotomine	Rodents, man	Americas	Rare

MENINGITIS

3. TTFFF
The specific clinical features of viral and bacterial meningitis in adults are indistinguishable on an individual basis: headache, malaise, nausea, vomiting, photophobia and nuchal rigidity are features of meningeal infection. Viral meningitis is however less severe. Clinical manifestations in children may be nonspecific comprising fever and irritability alone which makes differentiation even more difficult. Aetiological diagnosis depends on examination of the cerebrospinal fluid (CSF) and in particular the exclusion of bacterial and fungal infection. Typically, with viral meningitis there is CSF lymphocytosis (10–1000 cells/ml), a slightly elevated protein level and a CSF glucose concentration greater than two-thirds of that in the blood. Studies have however shown that 20–75% of patients will have a predominance of polymorphonuclear leukocytes on initial examination of the CSF. A repeat examination 6–12 hours later usually shows lymphocyte predominance. Also, meningitis due to mumps, LCM and enteroviruses have all been shown to occasionally reduce CSF glucose to well below 50% of blood glucose. Despite this, a CSF polymorph count of over 2000/ml, a very low glucose and protein concentration of over 2 g/l makes viral meningitis an unlikely diagnosis.

4. FTTTF
The specific diagnosis of viral meningitis, if attempted, is mainly directed at identifying enteroviruses and mumps. If specimens are taken early enough in the illness, the viruses can be cultivated from the CSF in cell lines (e.g. primary monkey kidney cells for enteroviruses, human embryonic kidney and Vero cells for mumps). Some coxsackie A isolates will not grow in cell culture but can be grown by intracerebral inoculation of newborn mice. Stool and urine culture for enteroviruses and mumps, respectively, are likely to be successful both early and late in the illness; although not necessarily diagnostic the presence of virus in these sites is strongly supportive of the diagnosis. Throat swabs may also be helpful and retrospective diagnoses can be made serologically by CFT or ELISA. Electron microscopy and immunofluorescence of CSF are not of value as the viral and cellular load is rarely high enough.

5. FFTFF
Lymphocytic choriomeningitis virus is an *Arenavirus* with a rodent reservoir. Humans acquire infection from infected rodents. The clinical picture is that of aseptic meningitis with 20% of patients having upper respiratory tract symptoms and signs. Diagnosis is usually confirmed by the detection

of a fourfold rise in complement-fixing antibodies although the virus can occasionally be isolated from the cerebrospinal fluid (CSF). Spontaneous resolution is normal but mortality has been reported. Herpes simplex viruses cause 0.5–5% of all cases of aseptic meningitis. This is usually in association with primary genital herpes so HSV-2 is most often responsible. Unlike HSV encephalitis, the virus can often be isolated from CSF. Recurrent meningitis has been recorded although spontaneous recovery occurs each time. Varicella zoster virus (VZV) can also be detected in the CSF of cases of aseptic meningitis associated with herpes zoster. Treatment for HSV and VZV meningitis with acyclovir hastens recovery from illness.

ENCEPHALITIS

6. TTFFT

Para-infectious (also called post-infectious) encephalitis is an inflammation of the brain that follows virus infection or vaccination. It is thought to have an allergic or autoimmune basis. Up to 20% of cases of encephalitis may be due to this phenomenon. It usually presents abruptly 4–14 days after viral illness and is clinically indistinguishable from true viral encephalitis. Recognized causes are measles (with a 10% mortality), varicella-zoster (less than 5% mortality), influenza and rabies vaccine. Measles is complicated by neurological disease in 1 in 1000 cases. Patients with para-infectious encephalitis almost always have a rash. Neurological sequelae occur in 20–50%. Adenoviral meningoencephalitis accounts for less than 5% of viral encephalitic disease. Serotype 7 is the commonest implicated and encephalitis is often part of systemic disease with pneumonia and hepatitis. The virus can usually be isolated from the CSF. Human immunodeficiency virus-1 (HIV-1) is frequently associated with neurological disease; in about 50% this is due to the effects of the virus; the rest are due to opportunistic infections and tumours. Dementia is the most commonly encountered manifestation but aseptic meningitis, myelopathy, pseudobulbar palsy and peripheral neuropathy have all been described. Enteroviruses cause fewer than 5% of cases of viral encephalitis and illness usually resolves completely. Meningitis is by far the commoner manifestation.

7. TTTTT

See Table 3.1

ENTEROVIRUSES

8. TTTTT

Enteroviruses can be distinguished from rhinoviruses by their acid stability and optimal growth temperature at 37°C. Currently there are five groups of serotypes recognised: (1) Echoviruses: an acronym for enteric cytopathic human orphan viruses. There are 31 types (echovirus 1–9, 11–27 and 29–33); (2) Polioviruses: three types (1–3); (3) Coxsackie A viruses; 23 types (A1–A22 and A24, no A23); (4) Coxsackie B viruses: six types (B1–B6); (5) unclassified enteroviruses: four types (68–71). Hepatitis A was classified as enterovirus 72 until recently. The viruses enter the body via the mouth and replicate locally and in the intestine. Excretion occurs in stools. Viraemia occurs as part of the infection. Immunity to any individual serotype is long-lasting. The viruses are resistant to detergents and can survive for several months at 4°C and years at -20°C. If associated with organic material such as food they can survive exposure to 60°C. They are however rapidly inactivated by 0.3% formaldehyde and 1000 ppm free chlorine.

9. TFTTT

Enteroviruses are associated with disease of many organ systems (Table 3.3). Despite replicating in the gut, case-controlled studies have not shown an aetiological association with diarrhoeal illness.

Table 3.3 Enteroviruses and associated diseases

Disease	Associated enteroviruses
Meningitis	All
Encephalitis	Echoviruses, Coxsackie A, Coxsackie B
Paralysis	All
Carditis	Coxsackie B, Coxsackie A, Echoviruses, Polioviruses
Pleurodynia	Coxsackie B, Echoviruses, Coxsackie A
Acute haemorrhagic conjunctivitis	Enterovirus 70, Coxsackie A24
Herpangina	Coxsackie A, Coxsackie B, Echoviruses
Hand-foot-and-mouth disease	Coxsackie A, Enterovirus 71
Boston exanthem	Echovirus 16
Other rashes	Echoviruses, Coxsackie A, Coxsackie B
Respiratory tract infections	All
Pancreatitis	Coxsackie B
Orchitis	Coxsackie B
Pyrexia of unknown origin	All
Chronic fatigue syndrome	Coxsackie B

10. TTTTF
Enteroviruses are responsible for the majority of cases of viral meningitis: 90% of those that have a diagnosable agent. Transmission is via the faecal–oral route and there is a strong association with poor personal hygiene. Most cases occur between 3 months and 14 years of age with a peak incidence in the summer months. The clinical picture of enteroviral meningitis is indistinguishable from that caused by other viruses with complete recovery being the rule. An exception appears to be cases that occur in children less than 1 year old where a significant number appear to have sequelae: impaired language development, lower IQ, small head circumference.

11. FTTFT
Polioviruses, as with all the enteroviruses, have humans as their only natural reservoir although the virus can be detected in faecally-contaminated environs. Transmission is predominantly faecal–oral with the point of entry being the oropharynx. Infection is asymptomatic in 90% but in cases of clinical illness there is an incubation period of 1–35 days (usually 2–3 days). In 4–8% of cases, an upper respiratory tract infection or influenza-like illness results. In 1–2% aseptic meningitis occurs and in only 0.1–2% will paralysis result. Paralytic poliomyelitis usually has an influenza-like prodrome before the onset of paralysis which may be spinal, bulbar or bulbospinal. Bulbar illness is commoner in children who have had previous tonsillectomy. This paralysis is due to destruction of anterior horn cells. It resolves in 10% of cases, leaves minor residual paralysis in 10% and serious disease in 80%. Diagnosis is clinical and supported by culture of the virus from stools (occasionally CSF) where it may be found for 3 months after the onset of illness. Treatment is supportive, including physiotherapy. The disease is not uncommon in developing countries such as India where wild-type strains are responsible. In those countries with high uptake of vaccine and good sanitation, most cases are due to vaccine strains.

MUMPS VIRUS

12. FTTTT
Mumps is a **Paramyxovirus** *and thus has a single-stranded negative-sense RNA genome, an envelope and surface glycoproteins with haemagglutinin function (in one protein) and fusion properties (on another in the case of mumps). There is only one recognized serotype. Transmission is thought to be via respiratory secretions as the virus replicates*

*in the respiratory tract and is shed in greatest numbers in these; droplet
and fomite transmission may occur. The virus is also excreted in the
urine in 75–100% of cases. An antibody response occurs within days
of infection and immunity is long-lasting although subclinical reinfections do occur. Immunity induced by vaccine strains is also in practice
lifelong.*

13. FTFFF

About 30% of primary mumps infections are asymptomatic. In symptomatic cases, after an incubation period of 12–25 days, the commonest
manifestation is parotitis. There is often a prodrome lasting up to
a week of fever, anorexia, myalgia and malaise. Parotitis is usually
bilateral and tender, with subsidence in a week. About 60% of individuals with mumps parotitis will have CSF pleocytosis although
only about 15% will have clinical evidence of CNS involvement
(meningitis, encephalitis, meningoencephalitis, Reye's syndrome).
Parotitis can also be caused by other viruses (coxsackie, echoviruses,
parainfluenza types 1 and 3, LCM, influenza A) some of which may
also cause meningitis. Mumps meningoencephalitis is associated with
the presence of virus in the CNS and if associated usually occurs
after parotitis; 1–2% of cases are fatal. Unlike uncomplicated mumps
infection which has seasonal peak incidence in the spring in temperate
climates, meningoencephalitis peaks in the spring and summer months.
Spontaneous recovery is normal but psychomotor retardation, deafness, hydrocephalus and paralytic disease have been reported. Other
complications of mumps infection include orchitis, pancreatitis,
endolymphatic labyrinthitis, migratory polyarthralgia, oophoritis and
myocarditis. Mumps orchitis has been described in 20–30% of post-
pubescent males but is rare before puberty when mumps infection usually
occurs. Spontaneous resolution occurs in 3–7 days although symptomatic
relief with non-steroidal anti-inflammatory drugs relieves the pain.
Testicular atrophy may occur but infertility and feminization are rare
phenomena. Oophoritis occurs in 0.5–7% of women but infertility does
not occur. Pancreatitis complicates 1–15% of infections and occurs days
or weeks after parotitis; one-third of cases do not have parotitis.
Adults are more likely to get this complication than children. Clinical
symptomatology is usually mild and complete resolution occurs although
diabetes mellitus has been thought to be a late sequela. Hearing loss
may be due to meningoencephalitis or endolymphatic labyrinthitis. The
latter is rare and leads to unilateral deafness.

HERPES ENCEPHALITIS

14. TTFFT

Herpes simplex viruses account for about 10% of all cases of sporadic (but not endemic) encephalitis. In neonates HSV-2 is the commonly associated serotype, HSV-1 in adults. HSV-2 infection has a worse prognosis and is more resistant to treatment. In adults 70% of cases are due to reactivation of latent HSV. The disease affects predominantly the frontotemporal areas of the brain bilaterally. A history of mucocutaneous HSV disease has been noted in 22% of patients with herpes simplex encephalitis but also with encephalitis due to other causes and is therefore not a useful diagnostic indicator. Similarly, 70% of neonates with HSV-2 encephalitis are thought to acquire infection from mothers who are asymptomatic. Neonatal herpes encephalitis is more common in premature infants and is clinically manifest at 1–3 weeks of age.

15. TTTTF

Herpes simplex encephalitis may have an acute or insidious onset and almost always presents with fever and headache. Behavioural and personality changes occur in 85% of cases, dysphasia in 76%, seizures in 67%, autonomic dysfunction in 60%, ataxia in 40% and focal neurological signs (hemiparesis, cranial nerve lesions) in 85%. There are also usually signs of meningeal irritation. CSF findings are variable but typically show a mild lymphocytosis, a few red cells, normal glucose and mildly elevated protein. Culture of the CSF is positive in 4% of proven cases. Approximately 3% will have no abnormal CSF findings. CSF anti-HSV antibody titres 20 times or greater than those in the serum is found in 40% (although this is also the case in 11% of biopsy-negative cases). EEG and CAT scans may show focal abnormalities and support the clinical diagnosis. The definitive diagnosis is made by examination of a brain biopsy for the virus. This has the added advantage of confirming alternative diagnoses (abscess, cryptococcal infection, toxoplasmosis, tuberculosis, tumour, etc.). In experienced neurosurgical units this procedure has a 1–2% mortality. In centres without such expertise, a trial of acyclovir is often used as a diagnostic test. Recent studies using PCR to detect HSV in the CSF are promising and may obviate the need for brain biopsy.

ARBOVIRAL ENCEPHALITIS

16. TFFTT

Arbovirus is a term applied to a group of over 250 enveloped RNA viruses that are transmitted by arthropods. They cause haemorrhagic fevers, rashes, arthritis, encephalitis and other infections (Paper 9). Endemic and epidemic infection occur. Worldwide, arboviruses are the commonest cause of encephalitis with Japanese B being the most prevalent. Clinically they are not reliably distinguishable so diagnosis usually rests on serology to detect antibodies (CFT, HAI and immuno-fluorescence). The viruses are uncommonly isolated from CSF or blood. Most infections occur in children. An inactivated vaccine for Japanese encephalitis B is now commercially available. Two doses given a fortnight apart in a month induce immunity in a month which lasts a year.

RABIES

17. TTTTT

Rabies virus is a member of the **Lyssavirus** *genus and* **Rhabdoviridae**. *It is enveloped with a characteristic bullet shape. There is a single-stranded RNA genome of negative-sense. The virus is rapidly inactivated at 60°C and is also susceptible to lipid solvents and detergents. Rabies infected animals have been found worldwide with the exception of some islands such as the UK where a 6 month quarantine of imported animals has prevented local animals becoming infected. Many warm-blooded animals can be infected by the virus: dogs, cats, bats and foxes are the commonest sources of human infection. Transmission to humans occurs principally by inoculation through the skin from a bite: the skin itself is a protective barrier. Airborne transmission from bats and laboratory contamination have been recorded but are rare. Human-to-human transmission has only been recorded via corneal transplants. Local replication of virus then occurs in subcutaneous tissue and muscle with subsequent spread to neural tissue where viral replication results in cytoplasmic inclusions called Negri bodies.*

18. TTTTF

Replication of rabies virus is slow and so the incubation period follow-ing infection is often several months. This incubation period is inversely related to the density of innervation of the bitten area. In general, children have shorter incubation periods than adults. It is this long incubation period that makes post-exposure prophylaxis feasible. Infection is often initially manifest as paraesthesiae at the site of bite, followed by headache, malaise, anorexia and nuchal rigidity. Progression to behavioural disturbance (agitation and aggressive behaviour) is accompanied in about 50% by 'hydrophobia', laryngospasm that occurs on attempting to drink. Some patients may have an illness resembling Guillain–Barré syndrome with ascending paralysis and areflexia. Finally coma and death result. The diagnosis of rabies is usually made on clinical grounds with detection of viruses in corneal epithelial cells or skin taken from the hairline by immunofluorescence as confirmatory tests; other tests are also available in specialist centres. CSF changes are unremarkable and serology is usually only helpful in cases that do not receive post-exposure immunization.

19. TFFFF
Rabies vaccines grown in human diploid cells and then inactivated have been available since 1976. They are highly immunogenic and 100% of vaccinees will have neutralizing antibody although booster doses may be needed after 2 years following pre-exposure prophylaxis. The vaccine is given into the deltoid muscle as a course of three injections of 20 IU/kg body weight; in the UK two doses are given 4 weeks apart with a third at a year. Local adverse reactions occur in up to 20% but the vaccine is otherwise safe. This and other vaccines have been used to vaccinate animal populations: for example, applying it to egg shells so that the shell causes inoculation via the oral mucosa. The management of rabies post-exposure consists of three main steps. The wound should be cleaned preferably with 20% soap or benzalkonium chloride solutions. Rabies immunoglobulin should be given, half into the bitten site. Rabies vaccination is then started and given as a course of five or six injections (on days 0, 3, 7, 14, 30 and 90 in the UK). The success of this regimen approaches 100%. A further component of management is the identification and destruction of rabid animals.

CHRONIC DEGENERATIVE DISORDERS

20. FFFTF
There are seven or more chronic neurological disorders of animals that are categorized because of their pathology as 'spongiform encephalopathies' (Table 3.4). They share the following properties: (1) rare, (2) long incubation period, (3) transmissible (experimentally, naturally or both), (4) non-inflammatory vacuolation of affected neurones, (5) presence of abnormal protease-resistant protein, and (6) no viruses have been implicated. One leading hypothesis is that an infectious protein, 'prion', which lacks nucleic acid is the causative agent(s). Kuru was a disease that occurred in the Faure-speaking tribes of Papua New Guinea but not elsewhere. It was associated with the cannibalism of dead relatives. The word 'kuru' means trembling and describes

prominent truncal ataxia that was characteristic of the disease. Since cannibalism has been discouraged, the disease has died out. CJD is a pre-senile dementia characterized by myoclonic jerking and rapidly progressive mental deterioration. It has been described in many parts of the world including the USA, UK and Central Europe. It usually presents after the age of 40 years with death occurring within 12 months. Diagnosis is dependent on the clinical features and brain biopsy. Sporadic and familial forms (GSS which is autosomal dominant) are recognized. Sporadic cases have arisen by transmission from donor organs such as corneal transplants.

Common presenile dementia or Alzheimer's disease is thought to have a strong genetic, not infectious, basis.

Encephalitis lethargica resulted in a condition, clinically indistinguishable from idiopathic Parkinson's disease, that occurred in young adults in association with influenza pandemics during the time of the First World War. Parkinsonian-like illnesses have also been documented following arboviral infections. No conclusive aetiological association has however been made between viruses and idiopathic Parkinson's.

There has been worry regarding the transmission of spongiform encephalopathies from animals to humans but there is currently no evidence of this.

Table 3.4 Sclerosing panencephalitis

Disease	*Natural host*
Kuru	Humans
Creutzfeld–Jakob disease (CJD)	Humans
Gerstmann–Straussler–Schinker syndrome (GSS)	Humans
Scrapie	Sheep, goats
Transmissible mink encephalopathy (TME)	Mink
Bovine spongiform encephalopathy (BSE)	Cattle
Chronic wasting disease	Deer
Unnamed	Ungulates

21. TFTFT

Subacute sclerosing panencephalitis (SSPE) is a rare degenerative disorder of the central nervous system. Eighty-five per cent of those affected are children between the ages of 5 and 14 years with the majority of cases occurring in white Caucasian males. The incubation period following initial infection with measles is from several months to many years with a mean of 7 years. It also occurs after measles vaccination although the risk is less than a fifth of that following natural infection. It presents initially as a non-specific illness with emotional disturbance, personality change and insomnia. Generalized and focal neurological symptoms and signs then follow. Dementia and death occur 6 months to 3 years after initial presentation. Diagnosis is based on characteristic EEG and CSF findings: raised measles-specific IgG in the CSF is almost pathognomonic. There is no treatment. The pathogenesis of the condition is complex and usually results from infection with a measles virus which is defective in its production of proteins, particularly the membrane protein M, and the immune response to these abnormal proteins.

RETINOPATHY

22. TTFTT
Herpes simplex viruses, varicella-zoster virus, cytomegalovirus, measles virus, herpes virus B and Rift Valley fever virus have all been associated with retinopathy in adults. The second of these is a particular problem in immunosuppressed patients and usually leads to blindness if left untreated. Rubella causes retinopathy as part of the congenital rubella syndrome. Herpes simplex virus and cytomegalovirus have also been associated with neonatal retinopathy.

DEAFNESS AND EAR INFECTION

23. FTTTT
Congenital hearing defects have been shown to arise from intra-uterine infection with rubella and cytomegalovirus. Acquired deafness has been caused by many of the viruses that are associated with meningo-encephalitis but in particular with measles, mumps and varicella-zoster. Sudden deafness following upper respiratory tract infection has also been reported but specific viral agents have not been identified. Similarly vestibular neuronitis, or labyrinthitis, is frequently associated with antecedent respiratory tract infection but a direct aetiological role has not been proven.

MYOPATHY

24. TFTTF
Influenza viruses can replicate in cultured muscle cells and clinical illness is associated with electromyographic features of myopathy. Influenza B has been recovered from muscle biopsies. Coxsackie B has also been isolated from the muscle of neonates with acute encephalomyocarditis;

and sero-epidemiological studies have supported their role in myositis, and myocarditis, in older children and adults. Ross River virus is a *Togavirus* that can cause epidemic polyarthritis. Some patients will complain of myalgia and *in vitro* studies have shown that the virus can cause muscle necrosis in mice. Tacaribe viruses are *Arenaviruses* that have mice as natural hosts. They are associated with haemorrhagic fever. Enteroviruses have also been considered as aetiological agents in chronic degenerative muscle disorders, such as polymyositis, but virus has not been detectable in muscle biopsies from these patients.

CHRONIC FATIGUE SYNDROME

25. TFFFF
Fatigue lasting 6 months or more is thought to affect 1 in 4 to 1 in 5 people in industrialized countries at some time. A number of specific fatigue syndromes have been described in the literature: myalgic

Table 3.5 Diagnostic criteria for chronic fatigue syndrome (*Ann. Intern. Med.* 1988; 108: 387–9)

Major criteria	1. New onset of persistent or relapsing dehabilitating fatigue, which decreases patient's daily activity to less than 50% of premorbid levels, lasting 6 months or more 2. Exclusion of other clinical conditions
Minor criteria: symptoms	1. Fever or chills 2. Sore throat 3. Painful cervical or axillary nodes 4. Unexplained general muscle weakness 5. Myalgia 6. Prolonged generalized fatigue after levels of exercise previously well-tolerated 7. Generalized headaches 8. Migratory arthralgia 9. Neuropsychological complaints 10. Sleep disturbance 11. Development of symptoms over hours to a few days

Minor criteria: signs
Physician documented on
  two or more occasions,
  more than a month apart
	1. Fever (37.6–38.6°C oral, 0.2°C higher rectal)
	2. Non-exudative pharyngitis
	3. Palpable or tender cervical or axillary nodes, ≥ 2 cm diameter

The diagnosis is made if both major criteria and eight minor (six symptoms plus two signs or eight symptoms) are satisfied encephalomyelitis (ME), benign myalgic encephalomyelitis (BME), Royal Free disease, epidemic neuromyasthenia, Iceland disease, Akureyi disease, chronic mononucleosis. These are probably all part of the same syndrome. In 1988 a case definition for chronic fatigue syndrome was introduced (Table 3.5). A number of agents have been considered as aetiological agents: Epstein–Barr virus (EBV), human herpesvirus 6, Inoue–Melnick virus, cytomegalovirus, *Brucella* spp., *Borrelia burgdoferi*, enteroviruses and human T cell leukaemia virus-1. Only the last two of these are still thought to be possibly linked; although EBV can result in chronic fatigue, large studies have not shown it to be consistently associated. Neuropsychiatric symptoms occur in about 70% of patients, as does a complaint of allergy to food or drugs. Immunological abnormalities have been described but no consistent pattern is seen. As there are no consistent physical or biochemical abnormalities there is no single test to confirm the diagnosis. Serological tests to detect recent infection with enteroviruses are often used to support the diagnosis but cannot be considered as more than this. The main differential diagnosis is from fibromyalgia. Management of the condition is supportive. Antidepressants, immunoglobulin, parenteral magnesium sulphate and Efamol marine have all had beneficial effects in some patients. Corticosteroids, acyclovir, liver extracts, folic acid and cyanocobalamin have shown no advantage over placebo.

MISCELLANEOUS CONDITIONS

26. TTFFF

Neuropsychiatric complications occur in 1–5% of hospitalized patients with EBV infection. The virus has been associated with encephalitis, aseptic meningitis, Guillain–Barré syndrome, optic neuritis, peripheral neuropathy, facial palsy, psychosis and depression. Depression following infectious mononucleosis is the most common. As virus is rarely isolated from the CNS in any of these conditions, the precise pathogenic mechanism is unknown. Reye's syndrome is a 'toxic encephalopathy' associated with fatty changes in the liver. Seventy-five per cent of patients have an antecedent respiratory tract illness and 15% varicella. A large number of viruses have been associated with the antecedent illness but the commonest are influenza (A and B) and varicella-zoster viruses. Cofactors such as salicylates and aflatoxins have been implicated: for this reason, salicylates are now rarely indicated for the management of childhood fever. Diagnosis is on clinical grounds. There is no specific treatment.

Progressive multifocal leucoencephalopathy is a demyelinating condition that occurs in immunosuppressed patients, either iatrogenically or by malignancy. It is thought to be due to the reactivation of a polyomavirus, JC, which is acquired in the majority of populations by the age of 50 years. The diagnosis is made by brain biopsy, usually at post mortem, but should be considered from the clinical picture and serological evidence of JC virus infection. (Detection of the virus in urine may also help.) The condition progresses rapidly but there are a few reports of recovery following treatment with cytarabine.

Demyelination and in particular multiple sclerosis has been associated with many viruses. Coronaviruses have been isolated from the CSF but have since been shown to be laboratory contaminants. Guillain–Barré syndrome is an acute inflammatory demyelinating polyradiculopathy which has followed many infections (both viral and otherwise). It is not uncommon affecting 1–2 per 100 000 in industrialized countries. The majority of cases have a prodromal viral illness and the strongest association is with herpesvirus infection. Diagnosis is on clinical grounds and is confirmed by examination of the CSF. This shows, typically, a slightly raised mononuclear cell count, grossly elevated protein levels and oligoclonal banding. Viruses such as enteroviruses and adenovirus-2 have rarely been isolated from the CSF. Spontaneous recovery occurs in 85%. There is no specific treatment. Viruses have also been associated with other acute neurological conditions: Kozhevnikov's epilepsy with toga viruses and measles and recurrent meningitis (no specific virus). These associations are unsubstantiated.

Paper 4 Viruses and the gastrointestinal tract

INTRODUCTION AND GENERAL PRINCIPLES

1. FTFFT

Diarrhoeal infection vies with respiratory tract infection as the major cause of death worldwide. It has been estimated that in one year, 1987–88, there were three to five billion cases of diarrhoeal illness and five to ten million deaths in Latin America, Africa and Asia. A significant minority (up to 40%) of cases do not have a defined aetiological agent but it is likely that viruses make up the bulk of these. The commonest identified pathogen in children under the age of 5 years is the rotavirus which is found in 35–52% of acute cases; it is responsible for 35% of those requiring admission to hospital. Viruses in general appear to play a more significant role in diarrhoeal disease in children than in adults. Although the majority of deaths due to virus diarrhoeal illness occur in developing countries, severe illness still occurs in developed nations. It is estimated that 110 000 children are hospitalized each year in the USA with 75–150 deaths. The elderly are particularly vulnerable to severe illness and fatality (85% of all deaths associated with diarrhoeal illness are in this age group). Persistent diarrhoea (defined as diarrhoea lasting 15 days or longer) occurs in about 1% of cases in developed countries. Most are due to bacterial causes but it has also been associated with rotavirus infection. It is a greater problem in developing countries where there is a significant correlation with premorbid malnutrition.

2. TTFTF

The virus most commonly implicated is the rotavirus. Other agents (enteric adenoviruses, astroviruses, caliciviruses) are less frequently found. Human enteric coronaviruses, toroviruses, pestiviruses and picobirnaviruses have been found in human stools but their role in causing diarrhoea is unclear. In case-controlled epidemiological studies, enteroviruses have not been shown to be a significant cause of gastroenteritis.

3. TTFFT

There are no specific antiviral agents available. Oral rehydration solutions containing glucose and electrolytes are all that is required in most cases.

The use of rice in these solutions has been shown to further reduce stool output. Bismuth subsalicylate has been shown to be beneficial in at least one study. Breastfeeding is a significant factor in preventing diarrhoeal illness but not in its treatment. Antibiotics only have a role in cases of superinfection with other agents.

4. TTTTT
The management of food-borne and nosocomial outbreaks have the same underlying principles. Apart from those already mentioned, other principles are: (1) bacteriological and virological investigations should be started at the outset, (2) cleaning and disinfection of infected areas with 10 000 ppm hypochlorite solution, (3) institution of enteric precautions, (4) case or cohort isolation of infected individuals, and (5) screening of asymptomatic patients, as well as staff, because asymptomatic excretion is common and may act as a reservoir. The use of 70–90% alcohol handwashing solutions has been shown to be beneficial in reducing cross-contamination. The mere act of handwashing is however probably more important than the agent used. The caliciviruses and astroviruses are very resistant viruses. For example, Norwalk virus retains infectivity at pH 2.7 for 3 hours, heating to 60°C for 30 minutes and treatment with 3.7–6.2 mg chlorine/litre. The latter are typical levels used in potable water treatment.

ROTAVIRUS

5. FTTFF
*Rotaviruses are ubiquitous agents that cause diarrhoeal illness in most mammals. They are members of the **Reoviridae**. Thus they are non-enveloped viruses with a capsid of icosahedral symmetry; this is double-layered with an overall virion diameter of 70 nm. Electron microscopy shows a characteristic 'wheel' morphology. The genome consists of double strands of RNA in 11 segments (other members of the family have only 10). As with influenza A, these segments can undergo re-assortment although unlike influenza new serotypes do not seem to appear. Also, unlike influenza A, animal strains of rotaviruses rarely infect humans (although canine and feline-related human strains have been noted in Japan). Each of these 11 genes encodes for a single protein, except for gene 11 which codes for two. There are four main structural proteins, with VP4 and VP7 on the outer capsid being responsible for the neutralizing immune response. At least seven different serotypes of rotavirus have been identified although most human infections are caused*

by serotypes 1–4. They can also be grouped on the basis of antigenic differences in the inner capsid protein; human pathogens fall into groups A, B and C. For epidemiological purposes further typing can be achieved by examining electropherotypes of the RNA segments. The viruses are relatively resistant to detergents, bile salts and ribonucleases which may contribute to their infectivity. Infection is limited to the mature enterocyte on the tips of villi in the small intestine with lysis of these cells and shortening of villi. Osmotic diarrhoea results from a lack of absorptive surface.

6. FFFFF

Rotaviruses are the commonest single cause of diarrhoeal illness worldwide; about 125 million cases and 800 000 to 900 000 deaths annually. They are more likely to result in hospitalization than other viral causes: rotaviruses account for 12–71% of all episodes in hospitalized children compared with 6–25% of mild diarrhoeal cases in the community. The peak incidence of rotaviral illness is between 3 and 15 months. Infants in the first three months of life are protected by maternal antibody. Severe illness is rare after the age of 3 years although adults may have mild illness. In most populations, 80% will have antibody by the age of 3 years. Transmission is mainly by the faecal–oral route although respiratory transmission has been suggested in volunteer studies. Rotavirus infections are commonest in the winter months in northern Europe and North America. In equatorial countries there does not seem to be a seasonal preponderance. Group A rotaviruses are most frequently found in North America and Europe, group B viruses are found mainly in China and group C viruses are worldwide but are infrequently found.

7. TTFFF

Rotavirus infections may be asymptomatic. It is not clear how frequent this is but it is not uncommon. Symptomatic infection is manifest as gastroenteritis that lasts for 5–7 days after an incubation period of 1–3 days. Characteristically there is frequent vomiting early in the illness and fever with a temperature of 38.5 °C or greater at some time during the illness. The diarrhoea is usually watery and often severe: the presence of bloody or purulent diarrhoea or tenesmus usually indicates concurrent bacterial infection. As part of the illness, metabolic acidosis may occur and be severe. Neurological abnormalities ranging from aseptic meningitis to subdural haemorrhage have also been recorded and are thought to be related to the metabolic acidosis. Respiratory symptoms occasionally occur but evidence for direct infection of the respiratory tract is lacking. Excretion of rotaviruses often persists after the period of illness but rarely for more than 8 days after the onset of illness, except in the immunocompromised who may excrete virus for 30 days or more.

8. TFFTT

The antibody response to rotavirus infections is predominantly serotype-specific although numerous studies have now shown that low-level heterotypic responses are common even after primary infection. Neutralizing antibodies are directed against the VP4 and VP7 proteins on the outer capsid. The level of protection against reinfection correlates roughly with the level of antibody response although reinfections do occur. Exogenous antibody, either in the form of colostrum or gamma-globulin, has been used successfully to abort infections. The diagnosis of rotavirus infections cannot be made solely on clinical grounds but is relatively simple as large numbers (10^{10} virus particles/ml in the first 2–3 days of illness) are shed in the stools and can be detected by electron microscopy. More rapid tests using latex agglutination and ELISA are also routinely used in many laboratories. Polyacrylamide gel electro-phoresis of RNA fragments is used for epidemiological purposes. Group A viruses will grow in cell culture (primary monkey kidney or LLC-MK2 cells) but this is not useful diagnostically. The management of infections is based on oral fluid and electrolyte replacement. Commercial prepara-tions are available. Zinc supplementation and colostrum given orally have been shown to have a role in cases of persistent diarrhoea. A number of different potential rotavirus vaccines have been developed. These include live animal rotaviruses, human–animal strain reassortants, attenuated human strains and genetically engineered VP4 or VP7 vaccines. None has yet been made available commercially.

ENTERIC ADENOVIRUSES

9. TFFFF

Adenoviruses of all serotypes may be found in stools but this is likely to represent gastrointestinal transit of swallowed respiratory pathogens. Two serotypes, 40 and 41, seem not to be associated with respiratory illness but with diarrhoea. They have been classified into a separate subgenus, F. Some studies have shown that enteric adenoviruses are second only to rotaviruses as a cause of paediatric viral gastroenteritis. They are responsible for 4–10% of all cases whether in the community or hospitalized. Approximately 2% of most populations asymptomatically excrete these serotypes. The incubation period to diarrhoeal illness is

8–10 days with watery diarrhoea appearing early. Vomiting usually follows the onset of diarrhoea. This lasts for 1–2 days but the diarrhoea lasts for 5–12 days. Dehydration and respiratory symptoms have been noted but are uncommon. Infants and young children are predominantly infected. Immunity following infection is thought to be long-lasting and reinfection rare.

10. FTFFF
The enteric viruses are fastidious and will not grow in cell lines used for cultivating other adenoviruses. They require specialized cells such as HEK, Chang or Graham cells. Thus presumptive diagnosis can be made by the detection of adenoviruses by electron microscopy that will not subsequently grow in routine cell culture. Confirmation of the 40/41 serotype can be made by immunoassays, nucleic acid hybridization or restriction enzyme analysis of the DNA. Specific treatment or vaccines are not available.

CALICIVIRUSES

11. FTTTF
The caliciviruses are non-enveloped RNA-containing viruses with characteristic morphology. They derive their name from the cup-like hollows (Greek, calyx*) that can be seen on the surface. The capsids are 27–40 nm in diameter and have knob-like capsomers. The RNA genome is single-stranded and of positive sense. From this a single struc-tural protein is produced; there is not an intermediate polyprotein cleavage step as there is with enteroviruses. There are a number of human pathogens which have been classified, or are likely to be, as caliciviruses. These include hepatitis E, human enteric caliciviruses, Norwalk, Hawaii, Snow Mountain and small round structured virus (SRSV) Japan 9. It is likely that most viruses currently called SRSV are caliciviruses. For convenience, we shall use the term 'human enteric caliciviruses of characteristic morphology' (HECVCM) of which there are five known serotypes.*

12. TTFTT
There are five recognized serotypes of caliciviruses which have been linked with winter vomiting disease and diarrhoeal illness. Two patterns of illness are seen with different serotypes being found in each pattern. The first is seen predominantly in children with diarrhoea in 96% and vomiting in 77%. The incubation period of this illness is 1–3 days and

it lasts 1–11 days during which virus can be detected in the stools. In the second pattern, there does not seem to be an age preponderance and the illness resembles that of the Norwalk agent (see 13) although epidemics are uncommon. Exposure to caliciviruses, as represented by detectable antibody, is far commoner than illness; 80% of 6–12-year-olds are seropositive.

13. FTFFT
Norwalk and Norwalk-like agents have until recently been thought to be distinct from caliciviruses. The main reason for this has been their less distinct surface structure under electron microscopy. Gene sequence analysis however shows gross homology with other caliciviruses. The Norwalk agent was first identified from an outbreak of gastroenteritis in Norwalk, Ohio, USA in 1968. Since then the virus has been found worldwide. About 40% of outbreaks of gastroenteritis involving cruise ships appear to be due to Norwalk virus. Transmission is usually by food (shellfish, salads, cake icing, etc.) and water; aerosol transmission has also been postulated. There appears to be a slight winter predominance although outbreaks occur throughout the year. Part of the reason for the large numbers affected is the high secondary transmission rate of 30%. Illness associated with Norwalk agents have been reported more commonly in older children and adults than in infants; this is despite studies showing that in the developing world 80% of 5-year-olds have antibody to Norwalk and that the peak acquisition of this antibody is between 14 and 36 months of age. In volunteers, immunity appears to last only a few months.

14. TTTTF
Illness due to Norwalk virus has been investigated in both volunteers and the outbreak situation. After an incubation period of 24–48 hours, vomiting and diarrhoea develop. This may be accompanied by headache and abdominal discomfort. The illness usually resolves in 24–48 hours although virus excretion in the stools may be detectable for a further 48 hours. Diagnosis is routinely made by electron microscopy of stools although other tests (IEM, RIA, ELISA, PCR) may be available in research laboratories. In an outbreak situation, CDC have developed diagnostic criteria which include: negative stool cultures for bacteria, illness lasting 12–60 hours, frequent vomiting and an incubation period of 24–48 hours. No specific treatment is available.

ASTROVIRUSES

15. FFTTT

Astroviruses are so-called because of their 'star-like' morphology although only about 10% of particles seen in electron microscopic preparations will be typical. They have been recognized in a variety of animals with diarrhoeal illness although there are no data on cross-species infection available. The viruses are non-enveloped with icosahedral symmetry. The genome is a single-strand of positive-sense RNA which codes for two or three major polypeptides. The viruses do not grow in cells routinely used in diagnostic laboratories but can be adapted to grow in LLC-MK2 and CaCo-2 cell lines. There are currently seven human serotypes recognized.

16. FTFFF

In volunteer studies the pathogenicity of astroviruses has been shown to be low. An incubation period of 1–4 days leads into 2–3 days of watery diarrhoea although occasionally it may be as long as 7–14 days. Accompanying symptoms may include vomiting, abdominal discomfort and general malaise. Although deaths have been associated with astrovirus diarrhoea, the illness tends to be milder than that due to rotaviruses. Children under 7 years of age and the elderly are particularly affected by astrovirus gastroenteritis with peaks of infection in the winter months. Approximately 70% of children have antibody to the virus by the age of 5 years in the UK. Recent studies have suggested that astroviruses may be more common causes of diarrhoeal illness than adenoviruses, causing up to 8% of cases of paediatric diarrhoea. Transmission seems to be by food (e.g. oysters) and water. Diagnosis is made by electron microscopy of stools; an ELISA is available in some centres. Management is supportive.

Paper 5   Viruses and the hepatobiliary tract

INTRODUCTION

1. FFFFF

Viral hepatitis was described in the writings of Hippocrates and has remained a major cause of morbidity and mortality worldwide. There are many viruses that have been associated with hepatitis (Table 5.1) but only those that have the liver as their predominant target organ are known as 'hepatitis viruses'. There are at least five of these (hepatitis A–E) viruses. They have common clinical and pathological features. They all cause jaundice, dark urine and pale stools and in most cases there are no distinguishing features. Pathologically the liver shows multifocal parenchymal cell necrosis and histiocytic periportal inflammation. Hepatitis A, B and C have been found all over the world. Hepatitis D was initially thought to be restricted to parts of Europe but has emerged in other parts of the world such as the USA and Australia. Hepatitis E appears to be more common in southeast Asia, China, North Africa, the former Soviet Union and Central America than in other parts of the world. The incidence of hepatitis B, mainly due to vaccination policies, is becoming less frequent in industrialized countries.

Table 5.1 Viruses associated with hepatitis

Common	Less common
Hepatitis A	Yellow fever
Hepatitis B	Epstein–Barr virus
Hepatitis C	Cytomegalovirus
Hepatitis D	Herpes simplex (types 1 and 2)
Hepatitis E	Varicella-zoster
	Rubella
	Ebola
	Marburg
	Rift valley
	Crimean–Congo haemorrhagic fever

2. TFTTF

The virus most commonly associated with acute pancreatitis is mumps. Less common are coxsackie viruses (particularly B1, B2 and B4), cytomegalovirus and Epstein–Barr virus. Coxsackie B virus has been implicated in the genesis of chronic pancreatitis and diabetes mellitus. Tataguine virus is an arthropod-borne virus found in West Africa. It is associated with a non-specific viral illness.

HEPATITIS A

3. TTFTF

Hepatitis A was originally classified as enterovirus 72 but has now been re-designated as a hepatovirus in the family **Picornaviridae**. *It is a non-enveloped virus of 27 nm diameter and a single-stranded RNA genome. Production of proteins is, as in other picornaviruses, by a polyprotein intermediate. Hepatitis A virus (HAV) is however significantly more resistant to denaturing agents than other members of the* **Picornaviridae**. *There is little loss of infectivity at temperatures up to 70°C or at pH 1.0 for several hours. It is also relatively resistant to enzymes such as trypsin. These characteristics must enhance its survival in faeces. Although only one serotype is recognized, at least seven genotypes have been defined. The majority of isolates from clinically ill patients belong to only two genotypes. The virus will grow, once adapted, in a number of cell lines but without much cytopathic effect. Wild-type virus is however much more difficult to cultivate and cell culture is not a useful diagnostic test routinely.*

4. TFTTT

Hepatitis A is found worldwide although there appear to be three broad patterns of illness:

(1) In developing countries where socioeconomic conditions and sanitation are poor, individuals become infected during childhood and 100% of adults are seropositive. Clinical illness is uncommon except in visitors. This pattern is seen in many parts of Africa, Asia and Central and South America.

(2) In the developed countries where sanitation and socioeconomic conditions are of a high standard, few children are infected and the incidence rises sharply in early adulthood to peak in the 30-year-old and 40-year-old age groups. This is the pattern in Europe and North America.

(3) This pattern occurs in countries where there is improving sanitation or where disease is no longer endemic but there is frequent re-introduction

of disease. Infection occurs in both childhood and adulthood. This has occurred in places such as Berlin in the 1960s.

Transmission is via the faecal–oral route with person-to-person spread being a significant feature. Outbreaks have also been documented from a large number of uncooked or poorly cooked foodstuffs: potato salad, cold meats, potatoes, custard, milk, shellfish and so on. They can also arise following contamination of foodstuffs after cooking. Water-borne outbreaks are relatively uncommon. In developed countries, hepatitis A is three times more common in young male homosexuals than age-matched heterosexual males. Transmission by blood products has been reported, presumably from donated blood collected from individuals in the viraemic phase. This is a rare phenomenon. The increased prevalence in drug addicts may be partly attributable to this but also to poor socioeconomic conditions. Virus has been shown to survive for several hours on the hands of inoculated volunteers which also raises the possibility of fomite transmission. In some parts of the world there is an autumn peak of incidence of infection. This has been found in Germany but not in the USA.

5. TTFTF

The incubation period is 2–6 weeks whether transmission is by the oral or parenteral route. Viraemia occurs throughout most of this period. In children anicteric infection is the rule with less than 10% under 6 years of age being jaundiced and 40–50% of children between 6 and 14 years of age. In adults 70–80% will become jaundiced. Initial symptoms are non-specific with fever, fatigue, headache, nausea, vomiting and abdominal discomfort predominant. Other symptoms occasionally occur: coryza, sore throat, diarrhoea, myalgia, rash. Immune complex disease is not a feature of hepatitis A infection. This prodrome lasts up to a week and heralds the onset of dark urine, pale stools and jaundice in that chronological order. In severe cases there may be systemic pruritus and abdominal pain. Icteric illness may last for a few days to several months with a positive correlation of length of illness with age. Chronic hepatitis lasting longer than a year is not common and may suggest co-infection with another agent. Relapsing hepatitis is however a feature. Acute fulminant hepatitis occurs in less than 1% with the majority of these cases being fatal. An increased severity of illness in pregnant women has been reported in Asia and the Middle East but not in the USA or Europe.

6. TTTFF

The detection of hepatitis A virus-specific IgM in serum by ELISA or RIA is the most reliable method of diagnosing acute infection with hepatitis A. It is almost always detectable at the onset of clinical illness and persists for 4–6 months, occasionally longer. Specific IgG is also present early during clinical illness and generally persists for life. Virus-specific IgA is produced both in the serum and as secretory antibody in saliva and faeces but is often undetectable in the first week of illness. The detection of virus-specific IgG or IgM in saliva appears to be more promising. Other tests have been used but not routinely. Viraemia occurs at the end of the incubation period and during early illness but detecting virus in blood is not reliable. Viruria also occurs but detecting virus in urine is also not a useful diagnostic test. Virus or viral antigen can be found in the faeces during the first week of clinical illness in about 50% of cases.

7. FFTTT

The management of hepatitis A is supportive and most will recover with bedrest. Only severe cases will need hospitalization. Strict isolation is not usually justified as the peak of infectivity has already passed by the time the patient is jaundiced and excretion of virus in stools decreases rapidly. Only small children who are faecally incontinent may merit isolation. Enteric precautions (1.12) are sufficient in most cases. The control of spread of hepatitis A from an index case in the community has up till now relied on the prophylactic use of normal serum immuno-globulin in close contacts; more widespread use may be justified in an outbreak. A particular problem is food handlers. They should refrain from handling food while shedding virus, usually for only a week after the onset of jaundice. Another group who have been given immuno-globulin are travellers from low to high prevalence areas. Low prevalence areas include North Western Europe, North America, Australia and New Zealand. Southern European countries such as Greece (but not Spain, Portugal or Italy), Africa, South America and most of Asia are high prevalence areas. As important as human-to-human transmission is food-borne transmission. Food, if properly cooked, should not be a risk. Steaming shellfish for 90 seconds or cooking to a temperature of 85°C for 4 minutes will inactivate hepatitis A virus.

8. TTFTF

Hepatitis A vaccines have been licensed in a number of developed countries. The first vaccine to be given a licence in the UK was a formalin-inactivated strain, HM175, which is grown in human fibroblast cells. It is given parenterally as two 720 unit doses 4 weeks apart. This results in a detectable antibody response in over 95% which lasts for over a year. A booster dose at the end of a year means that the antibody response remains detectable for many years. Antibody levels are higher than after administration of immune globulin for prophylaxis but less than after natural infection. The vaccine has few adverse effects. In the UK, it is recommended routinely for sewerage workers but not food handlers. It is also replacing immunoglobulin for travellers from low prevalence to high prevalence areas. It should however be noted that over 80% of cases reported in the UK have acquired their infection locally. There are no specific contraindications although it is cost effective to check for pre-existing immunity in those over 50 years of age as the vaccine is likely not to be needed. The cost of these vaccines is prohibitive for routine use in most of the developing world.

HEPATITIS B

9. FTTTT

Hepatitis B virus (HBV) is the prototype of the **Hepadnaviridae.** *It is the only member of this family which is a human pathogen but others cause hepatitis in animals (woodchuck, ground squirrel, duck) which have served as useful animal models for understanding hepatitis B infection. The virus is enveloped and contains a genome of partially double-stranded DNA. There are three important structural proteins: surface antigen (HBsAg), core antigen (HBcAg), and 'e' antigen (HBeAg) which can be detected in serum from patients. HBsAg is produced in great excess in natural infection which was useful for early vaccine development. The 'e' antigen is a subunit of the core antigen which forms the shell around the genome. A fourth protein, HBxAg, is thought to be involved in the genesis of hepatocellular carcinoma. The virus also codes for a DNA polymerase with reverse transcriptase function which is likely to be important in the integration of hepatitis B into chromosomal DNA – an initial step in carcinogenesis. Subtyping of hepatitis B is carried out for epidemiological purposes and has been based on antigenic differences in HBsAg. There is a common virus determinant, a, and two sets of mutually exclusive determinants, d or y, w or r. Thus subtypes can be adw, ayw, adr or ayr. Epidemiological mapping is better done by genome typing. Variants of hepatitis B have also been noted. These can be detected by testing for HBsAg but are not neutralised by standard anti-HBs antibodies and can cause infection in patients who have been immunized with current vaccine strains.*

10. FTTTT

Hepatitis B or 'serum hepatitis' is found globally although the prevalence varies. In industrialized countries such as the UK and USA it is less than 4%. In southern Europe it is 20–50%. In southeast Asia it is 70–90% in some countries. In southeast Asia the predominant subtype is adr while adw and ayw are common in the UK and USA. Since the advent of routine hepatitis B vaccination, the incidence in developed countries has fallen: there are now fewer than 300 reported cases per year in the UK compared with nearly 2000 in 1984 before the introduction of routine immunization. Most of the estimated 200–300 million carriers are in developing countries. The virus is found predominantly in blood but also in semen, vaginal secretions, saliva and urine. The concentration of virus in these fluids is less than that in blood. Thus those at 'high risk' are injectable drug users, recipients of unscreened blood or blood products, sexual contacts, infants of carriers, healthcare and laboratory workers. Inmates of custodial and mental institutions are also at higher risk. The mechanism of transmission to the neonate is thought to be by infected vaginal secretions perinatally but may also occur by breastfeeding or prenatally. Saliva and urine have not been shown to be significant sources of spread.

11. TFTFF
The clinical incubation period of hepatitis B is 2–6 months but HBsAg may be found in the first few weeks after infection both after blood transfusion and after experimental parenteral inoculation. This is evidence that liver damage is not entirely a direct result of the virus. Early symptoms are general and include fatigue and mild gastrointestinal symptoms. Classically, smokers begin to dislike the taste of cigarettes. In up to 10%, serum sickness occurs with maculopapular or urticarial rash, arthralgia, arthritis, polyarteritis nodosa, cryoglobulinaemia and glomerulonephritis. These features distinguish hepatitis B infection from other viral causes. Other possible immunologically-mediated complications such as myopericarditis, encephalopathy, polymyositis and Guillain–Barré syndrome have been reported but the aetiological association is unproven. Icteric illness occurs in about 50% of all cases of infection. Approximately 0.2–0.5% of these will develop acute fulminant hepatitis with encephalopathy, coagulopathy and metabolic abnormalities. Death ensues in the majority of these. Most cases of acute hepatitis B resolve within 4 weeks but 10% of adults will become 'carriers' with HBsAg persisting in the blood for 6 months or more; this occurs in >90% of neonates. The immunocompromised are at particular risk of persisting hepatitis B infection. There is also a slight male preponderance. About 50% of chronic carriers will have a mild illness, chronic persistent hepatitis, which resolves over a period of a few years. The other 50% will have more

severe disease, chronic aggressive hepatitis, which has a tendency to result in post-necrotic cirrhosis. It is thought that a fraction of these cases will develop hepatocellular carcinoma although cirrhosis does not seem to be a prerequisite for the malignancy.

12. TTTFF
In parts of the world primary hepatocellular carcinoma (PHC) is the commonest visceral malignancy. These are also the parts of the world where HBsAg-carriage is high: China, southeast Asia and sub-Saharan Africa. There are over 250 000 cases worldwide. PHC, like most malignancies, is likely to be multifactorial in origin but the evidence for hepatitis B virus being a major factor is convincing. Previous HBV infection is far commoner in patients with PHC than in the general population or other malignancies. Moreover, in HBsAg carriers PHC occurs 200 times more frequently than in non-carriers. A minority of cases of PHC are HBsAg-negative. Other initiating agents such as aflatoxin, alcohol and hepatitis C have been implicated in these cases. Woodchuck hepatitis virus also produces liver cancer in woodchucks and serves as a useful model for the human situation.

13. TFTFF
Figure 5.1 and Table 5.2 show the time sequence of hepatitis B markers and the interpretation of diagnostic tests, respectively. In general, the presence of HBsAg is diagnostic of the presence of virus and detectable HBeAg implies actively replicating virus and is a marker of higher infectivity. The presence of anti-HBc IgM suggests acute infection in the past few weeks. The presence of any antibody suggests recovery (or tendency towards that) from previous infection in the absence of an immunization history. These are detectable for many years. Not all tests are required in any specific situation. The finding of HBsAg in a patient with acute hepatitis who is unlikely to be a carrier is sufficient to make a diagnosis of acute hepatitis B; if necessary, this can be confirmed by the detection of anti-HBc IgM. The anti-HBs test is used as a screening test to check that immunization has been successful. An anti-HBs level of 10 IU/ml or greater is evidence of an adequate response to vaccine but most laboratories would recommend levels of 100 IU/ml to ensure continuing protection. It is also useful to know whether a carrier is HBeAg or anti-HBe positive as blood from the former is far more infectious.

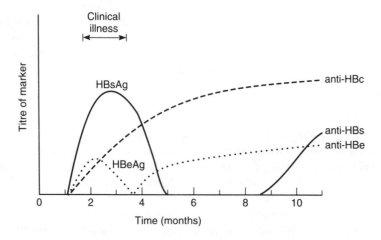

Figure 5.1a Time sequence of events in recovery from acute-hepatitis B.

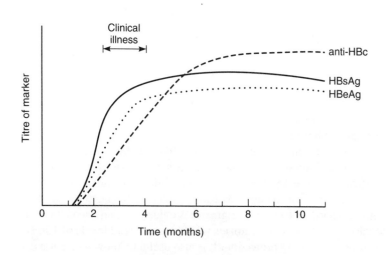

Figure 5.1b Time sequence of events in a hepatitis B carrier.

Table 5.2 Common hepatitis B marker profiles

HBsAg	HBeAg	Anti-HBc IgM	Anti-HBc	Anti-HBe	Anti-HBs	Interpretation(s)
+	+	−	−	−	−	Incubation period Early acute infection Infection with HBV variant
+	+	+	+	−	−	Acute hepatitis Carrier
+	+	−	+	−	−	Carrier
+	−	+/−	+	+	−	Carrier
−	−	+/−	+	+	+	Convalescence
−	−	−	+/−	−	+	Past infection
−	−	−	−	−	+	Previous vaccination Recent passive immunization Exposure without infection Previous natural infection
−	−	−	+	−	−	Previous natural infection False positive
+	+/−	−	+/−	+/−	+	Occurs in 10–30% with chronic active hepatitis

14. TFTTF

The management of uncomplicated hepatitis B infection is the same as that for other forms of viral hepatitis, namely bedrest. Management of fulminant hepatitis, whether due to hepatitis A or B virus, is also supportive and depends on close monitoring of clinical and biochemical status, particularly of encephalopathy. As hypoglycaemia occurs in liver failure, dextrose infusions are used. The withdrawal of exogenous protein, fluid control, vitamin supplements and avoidance of drugs are the other mainstays of management. A number of treatments have been tried in chronic hepatitis B: acyclovir, prednisolone, interferon inducers, arabinoside-A and derivatives and interferons. Only the last two of these, particularly alpha-interferon, have shown much promise. Favourable response (measured by clinical status, disappearance of HBsAg and appearance of anti-HBe and improved liver pathology) can occur in up to 50% of selected patients. Those most likely to respond are adult, Caucasian, heterosexual, within 2 years of acute infection and who are immunocompetent. The presence of active virus replication detectable by hepatitis B DNA polymerase assay and the use of treatment for at least 3 months also predipose to a favourable outcome. Relapse is however common in all patients. The use of an ancient remedy for jaundice, extract of a plant, *Phyllanthrus amarus*, has been reported as having a 59% success rate in eradicating HBsAg carriage but confirmation of this is required.

15. TFTTF
The standard procedures for preventing the transmission of blood-borne viruses apply to hepatitis B. These include the use of double gloves when handling uncontained potentially infected blood, screening of blood and blood products, the use of disposable or sterilizable medical equipment for use in invasive procedures, disinfection of contaminated materials and education of staff and patients. In addition, many centres have instituted screening programmes for hepatitis B, e.g. pregnant women.

Hepatitis B immunoglobulin (HBIG) is prepared from high-titre blood and is used for post-exposure prophylaxis. It is given as 300–500 IU intramuscularly within 48 hours of exposure. A second dose is often given 4 weeks later. Protective efficacy of this regimen has been calculated as 76% which may be improved to 90% with concurrent administration of vaccine. It should only be reserved for those who do not have evidence of pre-existing immunity to hepatitis B. Neonates born to infected mothers should also be given passive and active immunization.

Active immunization was first available with a plasma-derived vaccine is prepared from purified HBsAg from the plasma of carriers. In many countries this has been replaced by genetically-engineered vaccines. These are given intramuscularly as three doses at 0, 1 and 6 months. Seroconversion occurs in 95% of young adult immunocompetent women but in only 50–60% of immunocompromised patients. Alternative regimens have also been used. Intradermal vaccination is preferable in haemophiliacs although the seroconversion rate is marginally less. Short course regimens (e.g. 0, 1, 2 months with a booster at 12 months) also have advantages. Vaccination has until recently been prioritized to at risk groups in developed countries (5.10). Some countries, notably the USA and Canada, are now recommending universal vaccination in childhood. If facilities exist, evidence of seroconversion following vaccination should be sought 6–8 weeks after the last dose, particularly in those at risk of not responding. Antibody levels fall with time although the rate of fall varies from individual to individual. In those who adequately respond to a primary course, protective levels of antibody persist for 5–7 years. Boosters may be required at this time although there is little evidence to support the notion that falling antibody levels leads to a significant risk of reinfection.

16. TTFFT

A non-responder to hepatitis B vaccine is a vaccinee with an antibody level of less than 10 IU/ml. Poor responders are, arbitrarily, those who have an antibody level of 10–100 IU/ml. Non-responders tend to have one or more of the following features: obesity, be older than 50 years of age, immunosuppressed or on dialysis. Immunocompetent homosexual men also have a poorer response rate than expected and patients who are carriers will not respond. In all but carriers it is often worth repeating the course of vaccine but the majority will still fail to respond. There has been some success in this residual group using intradermal vaccination, but more immunogenic vaccines are likely to be a better solution. Poor responders will usually boost their immune response after further individual doses of vaccine.

HEPATITIS C

17. TTFTT

Hepatitis C is the virus responsible for the majority of cases of viral hepatitis that are not attributable to hepatitis A or B, so-called non-A non-B hepatitis (NANBH). The virus was first identified by infecting chimpanzees with material from infected patients. It is an RNA-containing enveloped virus of about 30–60 nm in diameter. The genome is 10 kb in size. It is a flavivirus although there are similarities with veterinary agents, the pestiviruses. It has been reported that the virus can be grown in T cell lines but this is not yet a routine method. The virus is found worldwide and there appear to be at least six genotypes. In the USA it has been estimated that 60–90% of NANBH post-transfusion hepatitis is due to hepatitis C; this is equivalent to 300 000 cases per year. Screening of blood donations has shown a 0.02–0.1% prevalence of hepatitis C virus (HCV) antibody in the UK. Like hepatitis B and other blood-borne agents hepatitis C is found more commonly in injectable drug users and haemophiliacs than in the general population. Both sexual and vertical transmission have been recorded but these are less common. HCV has been implicated in the genesis of PHC: 69% of Japanese patients with PHC who were seronegative for hepatitis B were HCV seropositive; this compares with 4–10% of a control population. The virus is not thought to contain an oncogene so an indirect mechanism is postulated.

18. TTFTF

An illness milder than hepatitis A or B occurs, usually after an incubation period of 6–9 weeks post-transfusion although periods from 2 weeks to 6 months have been reported. Fulminating hepatitis is rare. The most important distinguishing feature of hepatitis C is that over 50% of patients will become chronic carriers. About 20% of these will develop cirrhosis. Serum sickness is not a feature although mixed cryoglobulinaemia does occur. The diagnosis of hepatitis C infection can be made by the detection of antibodies. The first commercially available test was an ELISA that detected antibodies to the so-called C100 antigen of the virus. This appears to be relatively poorly immunogenic and antibodies are detectable only 4–32 weeks after infection. This is after the resolution of clinical illness. PCR appears to be able to offer a diagnosis of acute infection and antibody tests based on other antigens, such as C33 and C22, also hold promise. Management of chronic hepatitis C infection with alpha-interferon has been successful in 40–50% of patients. Liver pathology and function improve but relapse is high although there does not appear to be refractoriness to further use of the drug. Screening of blood by antibody testing prior to transfusion appears to be able to prevent the majority of cases of post-transfusion NANBH and has been instituted in the UK.

HEPATITIS D

19. FTTTF

Hepatitis D virus is a defective virus which requires another virus, usually hepatitis B (herpes simplex can play the same role in vitro), to replicate. It has a circular single-stranded RNA genome associated with a protein, known as the delta antigen, surrounded by a capsid of HBsAg. It is related to plant viroids. It is transmitted principally as a blood-borne agent although infection through open skin wounds (e.g. impetigo) from environmental sources has been recorded in children. Male-to-male sexual transmission is also documented. The virus has been found worldwide with prevalence in HBsAg carriers ranging from less than 2% in North America, northern Europe and Australia to 20–90% in the Amazon basin. The prevalence in southeast Asia is low.

20. TTFFT

Hepatitis D does not cause clinical illness in the absence of hepatitis B. It can co-infect, or superinfect a HBsAg carrier. Whichever scenario, the clinical presentation is of a more severe infection than that of hepatitis B alone. The risk of fulminant hepatitis is 10% in cases of co-infection and 20% in superinfections. Co-infection may also result in a biphasic illness in about 10% of cases. Although co-infection does not increase the chronic carriage rate of HBsAg, superinfection accelerates disease progression in carriers so that cirrhosis can develop within 5 years. Superinfection also results in chronic carriage of hepatitis D virus. The diagnosis of hepatitis D infection can often be made in the first 1–10 days of illness by the detection of delta antigen or later by the detection of antibodies. Although there is some evidence that interferon therapy and foscarnet may be effective in some cases of persistent hepatitis D infection and fulminant hepatitis, respectively, the mainstay of management is control of hepatitis B. Although hepatitis B vaccination will prevent co-infection, there are not any specific means of protecting HBsAg carriers from superinfection other than hygienic practice.

HEPATITIS E

21. TFFTF
Hepatitis E virus is a cause of enterically-transmitted NANBH. It is a small non-enveloped virus of 32–34 nm in diameter with a single-stranded RNA genome of 7.5 kb in size. It is most likely a calicivirus. Like other caliciviruses it is sensitive to freeze-thawing and high concentrations of salt. The virus has been associated with outbreaks occasionally involving tens of thousands of cases in India, central and southern Asia, former Soviet Union, North Africa and Mexico. It is often transmitted by contaminated drinking water.

22. TTTFF
Clinical illness caused by hepatitis E virus is indistinguishable from that due to hepatitis A. The incubation period is slightly longer and it is mainly adults between the ages of 15 and 40 years who become ill. In outbreaks recorded from many parts of the world, there has been a 10–20% mortality rate in pregnant women. In others, spontaneous recovery is the rule and chronic liver disease has not been reported. The diagnosis is generally by exclusion of other causes but can be confirmed by immune electron microscopy of stools. ELISA and RIA methods for antibody detection are in development. Management is symptomatic.

Paper 6 Viruses and the mucocutaneous system

INTRODUCTION

1. TFTFF

Viruses can cause a rash on the external body surface, an 'exanthem', and in some cases on a mucous membrane, 'an enanthem'. Strictly the former term is only applied to agents (infectious or toxic) that produce a rash through small vascular changes. Viruses that are typically associated with an enanthem are measles (Koplik's spots), rubella (Forchheimer spots), Epstein–Barr virus (palatal petechiae) and enteroviruses (various rash types). Papillomaviruses can cause lesions on any epithelial surface but the cutaneous wart is not strictly an exanthem.

2. TTTFT

See Table 6.1. Macules are dicoloured patches that are not raised; papules are small raised lesions. Papules become known as nodules when greater or equal to 1 cm in diameter. Vesicles are circumscribed elevated lesions containing clear fluid. Pustules are vesicles with purulent contents. Erythema multiforme begins as a maculopapular rash which develops into bullae (vesicles greater than 0.5 cm in diameter). It is recurrent and when associated with fever constitutes Stevens–Johnson syndrome. Herpes simplex (HSV) is the one virus that has so far been incriminated as an aetiological agent. HSV antigen, gB (a glycoprotein), can be detected in the lesion although infectious virus cannot be recovered. Moreover, there is strong genetic (HLA-DQw3 is a strong risk factor for herpes-induced erythema multiforme) and epidemiological evidence for the relationship.

Table 6.1 Viral skin rashes

Type of rash	Common viruses	Less common viruses
Maculopapular	Measles Rubella Parvovirus B19	Human herpesvirus-6 Enteroviruses Epstein–Barr virus Cytomegalovirus Hepatitis B Dengue Ross River Chikungunya Human immunodeficiency viruses Lymphocytic choriomeningitis
Vesicular/pustular	Varicella-zoster Herpes simplex-1 Herpes simplex-2	Enteroviruses Vaccinia Cowpox Orf
Nodular	Papillomaviruses Molluscum contagiosum	Pseudocowpox
Haemorrhagic	Dengue Hantaan Rift Valley Lassa fever	Marburg Ebola Crimean–Congo haemorrhagic fever Junin Machupo Others
Erythema multiforme	Herpes simplex	Epstein–Barr Adenovirus Coxsackie B5 Vaccinia

MEASLES

3. TTTTF
Measles virus is classified as a Morbillivirus, *in the family* **Paramyxo-viridae**. *The virions are enveloped, pleomorphic and 120–250 nm in diameter. The single negative-sense RNA genome codes for several proteins including a nucleocapsid (N), membrane (M), fusion (F) and haemagglutinin (H). Unlike other members of the family there is an absence of a neuraminidase. Infectivity of the virus is rapidly inactivated at 50°C, by acid pH and by ultraviolet irradiation. It survives storage at −70°C however for many years. There is only a single serotype although there are minor antigenic and genetic variants, particularly in the M protein. The natural host is man although primates can be infected.*

4. TTFTT

Measles is possibly the most contagious disease that infects humans. Within family groupings, 100% of susceptible contacts of an index case will become infected. Prior to the introduction of measles vaccination, epidemics occurred every 2–3 years which affected the vast majority of susceptible individuals. This high infectivity, coupled with humans being the only natural host, has made measles an eradicable disease. It has been calculated that at least 200 000 persons are needed in a community to enable continued transmission of the virus. Eradication has been recorded in some parts of the world but modern travel has resulted in continual re-introduction of disease. Transmission is by the respiratory route, probably by aerosols. Measles infection occurs worldwide but is now far commoner in developing than developed countries since the introduction of universal vaccination in the latter. Mortality is also much higher in developing countries particularly in children under the age of 2 years of age: 5–25% of hospitalized children in this age group still die. In developed countries, the introduction of measles vaccines has drastically reduced the incidence of wild-type measles infection. In the USA, 200–500 cases per 100 000 population were reduced to 1.5 per 100 000; in the UK the number of reported cases is now in single figures. In developing countries, children under 5 years of age are most commonly infected although not under 6 months of age because of the presence of maternal antibody. Seasonal peaks of infection have been reported worldwide: in temperate climates this is between February and April (in countries where infection is still common).

5. TTFTT

Measles is spread by respiratory secretions and patients were infectious as early as 3 days before the onset of symptoms and remain so till the rash desquamates. The illness is also known as rubeola and morbilli. The incubation period is 10–14 days during which virus may be detected in blood and leucopenia may be noted. The prodromal illness consists of upper respiratory tract symptoms and signs with progressive fever, which persist into the rash phase. Koplik's spots, clusters of bluish-white spots with secondary erythema opposite the upper molars, occur in 80% of cases during the prodrome. Resolution of Koplik's spots occurs in 48 hours and thus they may not be present when the exanthem appears. The typical rash begins on the neck near the hairline, spreads to the face and upper trunk, then the entire body surface over 2–3 days; an important diagnostic feature is that the rash stops at the hairline. There is a peak of fever on the second day of rash with subsequent defervescence. The rash fades over 4–5 days with desquamation insome cases. Respiratory symptoms are prominent and tend to resolve after the rash. A modified illness occurs in some children who have had previous immunization. There may be an attenuated illness or an uncommon syndrome known as 'atypical measles'. This latter syndrome occurred after the use of killed measles vaccine and is manifest initially as fever of sudden onset, headache, abdominal pain and myalgia. A rash then appears which starts on the distal extremities and then spreads to the rest of the body. It starts as maculopapular but may become purpuric or urticarial. The majority of cases then develop pneumonia with a significant mortality rate. Measles virus has not been isolated and an immunological basis has been postulated. Immunity to natural infection is lifelong in the absence of acquired immunosuppression.

6. TTTTT
The most serious common complication is secondary bacterial pneumonia. This is most commonly associated with *Streptococcus pneumoniae* and *Staphylococcus aureus* but reactivation of *Mycobacterium tuberculosis* has also occurred. *Neisseria meningitidis* is also a common secondary pathogen. Other complications include bacterial otitis media and subacute sclerosing panecephalitis (3.21). All complications are commoner in immunosuppressed patients. Infection in pregnancy is also associated with increased morbidity and mortality.

7. FFTTF
The presence of a typical measles rash with prominent respiratory illness (including conjunctivitis) does not require laboratory confirmation. If there is doubt about the diagnosis, virus can be isolated or detected by immunofluorescence from respiratory secretions for 2 days after the onset of rash and 4 days in buffy coat or urine. The rash is thought not to be due to direct infection but to be immunologically mediated. Retrospective confirmation of diagnosis can be made by the detection of a fourfold rise in IgG antibody by ELISA or complement fixation. Measles-specific IgG is not usually found in CSF except in patients with SSPE.

8. TTTTT
Inactivated measles vaccines have been replaced by live attenuated measles strains, typically Edmonston or Schwartz. In many countries they are now given with mumps and rubella in the MMR vaccine. As measles infection is usually acquired in childhood, for maximum effect the vaccine needs to be given as early as possible. The antibody response to vaccine is good with 95–100% efficacy. This response is also more

rapid than after natural infection and so the vaccine can be used for post-exposure prophylaxis if given within 3 days of exposure. Apart from patients suffering from tuberculosis there are no contraindications of use specific to measles vaccine. The principal adverse effect is febrile convulsions 5–11 days after vaccination which occurs in 1 in 1000 children. Human normal immunoglobulin can be used for passive immunisation in exposed immunocompromised patients.

RUBELLA

9. TFTTT
Rubella virus is classified as a Rubivirus *in the family* **Togaviridae**. *It is an unusual member of the family as there is not an invertebrate host. It is however an enveloped virus with a genome consisting of single-stranded negative-sense RNA. The virion has haemagglutinin proteins projecting through the envelope. There is only one major antigenic type although monoclonal antibodies can distinguish between, for example, wild-type and vaccine strains. Humans are the only natural hosts although subclinical infection can be induced in primates. Like other enveloped viruses, rubella is heat-labile and rapidly inactivated by detergents.*

10. TTTFF
Rubella is found worldwide although the age of acquisition varies markedly from locality to locality. In countries with routine vaccination programmes, a third of clinical cases are in adults; in other countries the peak age is in early childhood but cases still occur in adults. Peaks of infection occur in the late spring in temperate climates. Transmission is by respiratory secretions with 20% of susceptible contacts being infected after only brief contact. In families 100% of susceptible contacts will become infected.

11. TTTFF
Rubella generally causes a much milder illness than measles. Constitutional symptoms occur but are not prominent. Fever is present in about 50% of children but subsides within 24 hours of onset of rash. The rash starts on the face and spreads to the trunk; it is maculopapular but fainter than that of measles and fades in 1–4 days. Lymphadenopathy, particularly of the posterior auricular and suboccipital nodes, is a feature of rubella; it may be present without the rash. Complications include encephalitis, thrombocytopenia, leucopenia and arthritis. Acute polyarthritis affecting small and medium-sized joints occurs most

commonly in post-pubertal females. It usually resolves spontaneously over a period of weeks although, rarely, chronic arthritis has been reported. Leucopenia and thrombocytopenia are common but not usually of clinical significance. Purpura and haemolysis occur rarely. These haematological problems are thought to have an immunological basis. Rubella infection usually leads to long-lasting immunity but reinfections occur in 1.5–4%. These tend to be subclinical but when clinically apparent in pregnant women may lead to teratogenicity and fetal loss (6.12).

12. TTTTF

Table 6.2 Manifestations of congenital rubella syndrome

General	Low birth weight
	Growth retardation
	Psychomotor retardation
	Behavioural and psychiatric disorders
	'Failure to thrive'
Cardiovascular	Patent ductus arteriosus
	Pulmonary artery stenosis
	(septal defects, coarctation of the aorta, aortic stenosis, myocarditis less common)
Eye	Microphthalmia
	Glaucoma
	Cataracts
	'Salt and pepper' retinopathy
Ear	Bilateral sensorineural deafness
Others	Thrombocytopenia
	Haemolytic anaemia
	Hepatosplenomegaly
	Hepatitis
	Pneumonia
	Encephalitis
	Post-rubella panencephalitis
	'Celery-stalk' bones
	Diabetes mellitus
	Thyroid dysfunction

Congenital rubella syndrome (CRS) was first described by the Australian ophthalmologist, Norman Gregg, in 1941. He described a syndrome of congenital cataracts, heart defects and low birth weight. Many other manifestations have since been recognized (Table 6.2). CRS and spontaneous abortion occur with primary maternal infection in the first 4 months of pregnancy. If infection occurs in the first month it has been reported that spontaneous abortion or CRS occurs in 61%, in the second month 26% and 8% in the third month; some recent data have however suggested that the risks are higher. Because of this, high risk termination is usually recommended. CRS has a mortality of 10–15% within the first year.

13. TFTTF

The diagnosis of rubella infection outside the neonatal period is usually made on clinical grounds but can be confirmed by the detection of virus-specific IgM or a fourfold rise in IgG antibodies. IgM is usually detectable at the onset of illness and persists for 1–3 months or longer. Most laboratories use an IgM capture radioimmunoassay (MACRIA) or enzyme immunoassay (MACELISA). The laboratory is more commonly involved in determining immune status. In the UK and Scandinavia this is done by means of single radial haemolysis (SRH). The presence of 15 IU/ml or greater is taken as evidence of immunity but lower levels may still confer adequate protection. In the USA, haemagglutination-inhibition (HAI) and ELISA are preferred. Both these test formats are more sensitive than SRH. Presence of antibody detected by these tests but not by SRH suggests early infection. HAI titres of 1 : 8 or greater are detectable at the onset of rash and persist for life; there is, however, usually an eightfold loss of titre 20 years after infection. A specific diagnostic dilemma is that of reinfections as most are subclinical. If serum is available from a time prior to exposure then a fourfold rise in IgG antibody is diagnostic. Alternatively specific IgM may be found. Some centres report the use of rubella-specific antigen–antibody avidity assays as helpful; these are not however widely available. The diagnosis of CRS is supported by culture of virus from infected organs, urine and pharyngeal secretions and by the detection of rubella-specific IgM in cord blood.

14. FTTTF

Universal vaccination for rubella was introduced in the USA in 1969 but in the UK a selective policy of vaccinating only pre-pubertal females was used. With the advent of the MMR vaccine, universal vaccination is now normal. Rubella vaccines are live attenuated Cendehill or RA27/3 strains. They result in seroconversion in 95% of vaccinees. Contraindications include immunosuppression and pregnancy although no cases of CRS have been reported from inadvertent administration of rubella vaccine in pregnant women. In general however women should take precautions to avoid pregnancy for a month after vaccination. Adverse effects have been reported in 10–15% of vaccinees: mild rubella, arthralgia and arthritis and peripheral neuropathy occur at differing intervals post-vaccination. Reinfections are also more frequent after vaccination than after natural infection occurring in 4–60%. These are subclinical in the vast majority with low teratogenic potential.

PARVOVIRUS B19

15. FFTFT
Human parvovirus B19 belongs to the genus Parvovirus *of the family* **Parvoviridae.** *Unlike other members of the family, (the dependoviruses which include adeno-associated viruses found in humans but apparently not pathogenic), paroviruses are not defective. B19 is a naked icosahedral virus containing a single strand of DNA. Infectious particles contain positive-sense DNA; complementary sense DNA can be found in other particles. The viruses are relatively resistant to lipid detergents and heat but not extremes of pH B19 has a tropism for erythroid progenitor cells* in vivo *but* in vitro *culture has proved difficult. Its effect on erythroid and other mitotically-active cells is to lyse them.*

16. FFTFF
B19 has been found worldwide with the normal age of acquisition being at 4–10 years of age. Incidence of infection is commoner during the late winter to early summer months in temperate climates with 3–5 year cycles of peak occurrence. Transmission is predominantly by the respiratory route although transmission by blood and blood products has been recorded. The incubation period is 6–11 days.

17. TTTTT
The majority of infections with B19 are missed or subclinical as 60% of young adults are seropositive. The commonest clinical presentation is erythema infectiosum (also called fifth disease and 'slapped cheek syndrome') which is seen as fever and a maculopapular rash in children. There may be mild, short-lived prodromal symptoms of malaise, myalgia, headache and chills which occur several days before the rash. The typical rash starts as erythema on the face (the 'slapped cheeks') which may spread to the trunk and limbs over 1–4 days. It may persist for 1–43 weeks with fluctuation of prominence. Adults are less likely to get a rash but are more likely, particularly women, to suffer arthropathy; this occurs in up to 80% of women with rash. Recovery from the illness may take 4 weeks or more. Aplastic crises occur in some patients

with chronic haemolytic anaemia, such as sickle cell or betathalassaemia. Patients with leukaemia undergoing chemotherapy may also suffer aplastic crises. Supportive therapy is required until infection subsides. Infection in the second trimester of pregnancy is associated with hydrops fetalis, which may result in fetal death. Infection in the first trimester has been associated with a marginal increase in the rate of fetal loss. Other reported complications of B19 infection include purpura, leucopenia, nephropathy and hepatitis. Chronic B19 infection with aplasia has also been reported in immunocompromised patients. The diagnosis of B19 infection can be confirmed by detection of virus-specific IgM (by MACRIA or ELISA). There is no specific treatment although immune globulin has been successful in the eradication of chronic infection in the immunocompromised.

HUMAN HERPESVIRUS-6

18. TTFTF
Human herpesvirus-6 (HHV-6) was originally found in lymphocytes from patients with lymphoreticular disorders. It has since been found in the general population. Putatively it has been classified in the herpes subfamily **Betaherpesvirinae** *because of its relatedness to cytomegalovirus. It can be grown in suspended cell culture (T lymphocyte cell lines) although not in cell monolayers. It is thought to be transmitted by saliva in the first few years of life; 60% of 1-year-olds have antibody to HHV-6. There is no evidence of sexual transmission.*

19. TFTFF
There is now a great body of evidence implicating HHV-6 as the cause of roseola infantum (also known as exanthem subitum). This is characterized by the sudden onset of fever which abruptly subsides in 3–5 days to be followed by a macular rash that starts on the neck and upper trunk. The rash then spreads to the rest of the trunk, limbs and less commonly to the face. It fades within 1–2 days with minimal desquamation. A minority of patients may have abdominal or upper respiratory tract symptoms. It usually affects children between 4 months and 2 years of age although children up to 5 years of age are affected. Outbreaks have been recorded with a case-to-case interval of 5–15 days. There is no seasonal predominance. Fatal hepatitis and haematophagocytic syndrome have also been recorded with HHV-6 infection. Association with lymphomas, post-viral fatigue and progression of AIDS have been noted but an aetiological role is unsubstantiated. The diagnosis of

HHV-6 infection is not routinely made. In specialist laboratories, virus and antibody can be detected in saliva by immunofluorescence. The detection of both HHV-6-specific IgG and IgM in the serum may be due to reactivation of latent virus; this also occurs with primary EBV and CMV infections. Specific treatment and vaccines are not yet available.

VARICELLA-ZOSTER VIRUS

20. TTTTT
Varicella-zoster virus (VZV) is related to the herpes simplex viruses and shares one or more antigens with them. This may result in a cross-reactive serological anamnestic response. It also exhibits latency in neural tissue. There are also significant differences in that it does not, for example, possess a thymidylate kinase although it does possess a thymidine kinase. Several gene types can be identified but there is only one major serotype.

21. TTFTF
VZV infection and chickenpox are common worldwide. Chickenpox is a highly infectious disease with secondary attack rates of 80–90%. Most cases occur in children between 3 and 9 years of age in temperate climates: 97.5% of young adults are seropositive in the USA. In tropical areas, such as parts of India, the disease mainly affects young adults. Transmission is by the respiratory route. The incidence of chickenpox, but not herpes zoster, peaks during the winter months.

22. TTFTF
VZV causes a primary infection, chickenpox, but may reactivate to produce herpes zoster (6.23). There is often a short prodrome of 24–48 hours, particularly in adults, of malaise and fever before the onset of rash. The rash begins as a maculopapular rash on the face and rapidly progresses to vesicles and pustules and spreads to the trunk and limbs. New lesions appear over 3–7 days. This 'cropping' is a diagnostic feature of chickenpox. The rash finally scabs but scarring is unusual in the absence of secondary infection. The rash may be atypical in areas covered by clothing or on eczematous skin; cropping may be absent. Complications occur more commonly in adults than children and with greater severity in patients with defective cell-mediated immunity. Encephalitis, pneumonia and bacterial superinfection are the commoner complications. About 15% of adults will develop pneumonia. Most will recover with the exception of pregnant women who have a 15–45% mortality

if left untreated. Encephalitis occurs infrequently (about one to two cases per 10 000 with chickenpox) but VZV is still in the three most common identified causes in temperate climates. Mortality is 10–15%. Other reported complications include transverse myelitis, meningitis, acute cerebellar ataxia, optic neuritis, Guillain–Barré syndrome, Reye's syndrome, ophthalmoplegia, carditis, pericarditis, parotitis, laryngitis, arthritis, coagulopathy, orchitis, glomerulonephritis and hepatitis. Many of the latter diseases in this list may well be chance associations. Varicella infection in pregnancy causes a significant risk of mortality for the mother. If acquired in the first 20 weeks it may rarely cause the congenital varicella syndrome (scarring of the skin, limb hypoplasia, cataracts, retinitis and psychomotor retardation). If it occurs late in pregnancy, neonatal varicella may result. Disease in the neonate is far less likely if the onset of disease in the mother is 8 days or more before delivery because of the transfer of maternal antibodies.

23. TTTTT
Reactivation of VZV to produce herpes zoster can occur at any age although the vast majority occur in adults over the age of 50 years. There may be a prodrome lasting several weeks (but shorter duration of dermatomal or visceral pain), followed by a rash which is classically dermatomal but may be generalized with lymphadenopathy (a few extra-dermatomal spots are common even in delineated rashes). If reactivation of virus has occurred from sacral ganglia, dysuria, polyuria, urinary retention or impotence may occur. Zoster affecting the ophthalmic branch of the trigeminal nerve may lead to conjunctivitis and keratitis. The most common complication is post-herpetic neuralgia. This virtually never occurs in children but persists for over 6 months in 25% of elderly patients. Other complications include facial palsy, Guillain–Barré syndrome, myelitis and meningoencephalitis. Herpes zoster in pregnancy has a benign prognosis for mother and fetus.

24. FTFTF
The characteristic rash of chickenpox and the dermatomal distribution of herpes zoster are usually sufficient to make a diagnosis. Confusion may rarely arise with herpes simplex and enteroviruses which may produce both varicelliform and zosteriform lesions. In such cases, VZV can be isolated from vesicles and will produce cytopathic effects in 3–8 days although as long as 21 days may lapse. Detection of a fourfold rise in antibody is often used to back up the diagnosis. The presence of a high titre of complement fixing antibody may also confirm infection as this antibody does not persist; caution should be taken however

as there is cross-reactivity with HSV. Specific IgM can be detected up to 3 months after infection and is particularly useful in cases of neonatal varicella. Screening for VZV-specific antibody in healthcare workers and high-risk patients (e.g. those with cancer) minimizes the problems of nosocomial infection. Nevertheless, 80% of individuals who do not give a history of having had chickenpox will be seropositive.

25. TTTTT

In most patients the management of infection with VZV is symptom-based, e.g. calamine lotion for pruritus. In the immunocompromised and pregnant women more active management may be required. Zoster immune globulin (ZIG) is prepared from blood donors who give a history of recent chickenpox or herpes zoster. It is given to immunosuppressed patients (particularly those with lymphoreticular disorders), pregnant women and 'at risk' infants who have been in contact with chickenpox. It needs to be given within 10 days of exposure, the sooner the better. Acyclovir is indicated for serious complications of infection. It is used topically or orally in patients with ophthalmic zoster. It improves the resolution of pneumonia in both pregnant women and other adults. Although some studies have shown a reduction in the incidence and severity of post-herpetic neuralgia, this is not yet an accepted indication. Higher doses of acyclovir need to be used than for the treatment of herpes simplex infections. The OKA strain of VZV has been shown to confer useful protection in immunocompromised patients but is not yet licensed in the USA or UK. It produces seroconversion in 70–90% of recipients with antibody persistence for 6–10 years. Other remedies such as capsaicin, psychotherapy and acupuncture have had reported success in the cessation of post-herpetic neuralgia but large placebo-controlled studies have not yet been carried out.

POXVIRUSES

26. TFTFF

There are at least two genera of poxviruses that have members infecting humans (Table 6.3). Smallpox (variola) was officially eradicated in 1979. Vaccinia is a laboratory strain of cowpox used as a vaccine for smallpox and is still used as a vehicle for potential vaccines. Apart from a mild smallpox-like illness that occurs rarely in vaccinees, particularly those with skin disorders ('eczema vaccinatum'), these two viruses are no longer of great medical interest. Poxviruses are the largest viruses that infect humans and are characterized by their size (160–250 × 250–300 nm) and brick-shaped morphology. They possess an envelope which encloses a central dumbell-shaped core, called a nucleoid, either side of which is a lateral body. Parapoxviruses are thinner than orthopoxviruses. The DNA genome codes for over 100 polypeptides. Unusually for a DNA virus, replication takes place entirely in the cytoplasm of infected cells although nuclear factors are involved. All the viruses can be grown either on cell monolayers or chick allantoic membrane, except molluscum contagiosum. They are relatively resistant to disinfectants, heat and drying.

Table 6.3 *Poxviruses pathogenic to humans*

Genus	Virus	Animal host(s)	Epidemiology
Orthopoxvirus	*Cowpox*	*Cattle* *Cats* *?Rodents* *?Elephants*	*Europe*
	Monkeypox	*Monkeys* *Squirrels*	*West and Central Africa*
	Vaccinia		*Laboratories*
	Variola		*Eradicated*
Parapoxvirus	*Orf*	*Sheep* *Goats*	*Worldwide*
	Pseudocowpox	*Cattle*	*Worldwide*
Unclassified	*Mollusum contagiosum*	*Man*	*Worldwide*

27. TTFFF

Cowpox appears to be confined to the UK and continental Europe. It is rare even in these areas. Although it was first reported in cattle workers, most cases have been without contact with cattle. Rodents and cats may be more important reservoirs. The rash usually begins as papules which become nodulo-vesicular and haemorrhage. These are painful. It is usually confined to the hands but may be self-transferred to the face. Systemic features (lymphadenopathy, fever and malaise) occur particularly in children and the patient may require hospitalization. Spontaneous resolution occurs in 4–6 weeks. Diagnosis is made on clinical grounds but can be confirmed by either electronmicroscopy of lesion extracts or growth of virus. Severe cases respond to anti-vaccinia immunoglobulin. Steroids exacerbate symptoms and methisazone, which has been used successfully in cases of vaccinia, is unhelpful. Pseudocowpox and orf have minor genomic differences but are principally differentiated on the basis of whether the virus was acquired from cattle or sheep (or their respective meat products). About 1–2% of abattoir workers are affected in any one year. A painless granulomatous lesion occurs on the hands without constitutional symptoms; spontaneous resolution tends to occur in a few weeks but reinfection is not uncommon. Idoxuridine has been successfully used to accelerate healing. Erythema multiforme has been reported as a complication but most infections are trivial. Monkeypox is a zoonosis with human-to-human transmission, albeit uncommonly. The clinical illness is a rash that appears on the face and spreads to the trunk. The lesions are like those of chickenpox including cropping and lymphadenopathy. The vast majority of cases have occurred in children with a 10–15% mortality. A vaccine is available for use in endemic areas. Tanapox produces a short prodromal illness of fever, headache and backache which is followed by the appearance of one or two papules on the trunk, face or arms. These papules become vesicular and umbilicated. Spontaneous resolution occurs. Diagnosis is on clinical grounds in travellers from endemic areas and can be confirmed by electron microscopy or culture of lesions.

MISCELLANEOUS

28. FFTFF
Kawasaki syndrome is an acute febrile exanthematous disease of children. Features of the illness are fever, conjunctivitis, oral changes (red, cracked lips, 'strawberry tongue' and generalized erythema), generalized urticarial or maculopapular rash and unilateral cervical lymphadenopathy. Oedema, erythema and peeling of the skin and hands are also diagnostic features. Almost all patients have CNS disturbance with irritability, lethargy, meningism or coma. Diarrhoea, abdominal pain, urethritis and hepatitis occur in 20–70%. About half also have cardiac abnormalities, the principal cause of the fatalities which occur in 2% of all cases, including myocarditis, coronary artery aneurysms, infarction and ECG aberrations. Arthritis is seen in 35–40%. Epidemics have been reported which suggest an infectious aetiology but no single agent has been consistently implicated. Supportive therapy is required for complications. Aspirin and gamma-globulin are the mainstay of general management.

Q fever is an acute febrile illness, often with atypical pneumonia. It is due to a Rickettsia. Patients with a rare inherited condition, epidermodysplasia verruciformis, develop squamous cell carcinoma after infection with papillomaviruses. Eczema vaccinatum is a generalized vesicular rash occurring in patients with underlying eczema. It occurs after administration of vaccinia. A similar rash, eczema herpeticum, occurs with herpes simplex virus infection. About 3–5% of patients with uncomplicated infectious mononucleosis develop a maculopapular rash (10.3).

Paper 7   Viruses and the genitourinary tract

INTRODUCTION

1. TFTTT
Many viruses can be transmitted by sexual activity (Table 7.1). Only four viruses however commonly cause lesions of the genital tract: herpes simplex types 1 and 2, molluscum contagiosum and genital papillomaviruses.

Table 7.1 Viruses transmitted by sexual activity

Route	Virus
Major route of transmission	Human immunodeficiency virus-1
	Human immunodeficiency virus-2
	Hepatitis B
	Herpes simplex virus-2
	Herpes simplex virus-1
	Human papillomaviruses 6, 11, 16, 18 (and others)
	Molluscum contagiosum
	Cytomegalovirus
Minor route of transmission	Hepatitis D
	Hepatitis C
	Hepatitis A
	Polioviruses
	Epstein–Barr virus
	Adenoviruses 19, 21, 34, 35, 37
Rare route of transmission	Marburg
	Ebola

2. TTFTT
See Table 7.2.

Table 7.2 Viral infections of the genitourinary tract

Disease	Virus
Genital ulcer	Herpes simplex-2
	Herpes-simplex-1
Genital warts	Papillomaviruses 6, 11, 16, 18
	Molluscum contagiosum
Vaginitis/vulvitis	Herpes simplex-2
	Herpes simplex-1
Balanitis	Herpes simplex-2
	Herpes simplex-1
Urethritis	Herpes simplex-2
	Herpes simplex-1
	Adenovirus 37
Cervicitis	Herpes simplex-2
	Herpes simplex-1
	Adenovirus 37
Cystitis	Cytomegalovirus
Acute haemorrhagic cystitis	Adenovirus 11, 21
Nephropathy	Cytomegalovirus
	Hantaan
	Hepatitis B
	Puumula
	B19 (one case)
Haemolytic-uraemic syndrome	Enteroviruses
Orchitis	Mumps
	Coxsackie B
Epididymitis	Mumps
Oophoritis	Mumps
Genital cancer	Human papillomaviruses

HERPES SIMPLEX VIRUSES

3. TTTTF
A virus is included in the **Herpesviridae** *on the basis of the four morphological features. There are seven recognized human herpesviruses (Table 7.3) which are grouped into three subfamilies on the basis of biological properties.* **Alphaherpesvirinae** *exhibit a variable host range, relatively short replicative cycle, spread rapidly in cell culture, destroy infected cells and exhibit latency in sensory ganglia. Infection occurs by direct inoculation of skin or mucosa where it causes local disease. The virus then tracks*

up sensory nerves to a sensory ganglion where it becomes latent in neurones (VZV in satellite cells). Under the influence of certain stimuli, the virus can then track down the nerve to cause recurrent infection. This is a very simple model but suffices for the purpose of understanding latency. **Betaherpesvirinae** *have a restricted host range, long replicative cycle and spread slowly from cell to cell. Latency is maintained in lymphoreticular (and other) cells.* **Gammaherpesvirinae** *have a limited host range, replicate in lymphoblastoid cells and may cause lytic infection.*

Table 7.3 *Herpesviruses that infect humans*

Subfamily	Genus	Virus	Common name
Alphaherpesvirinae	*Simplexvirus*	*Human herpesvirus-1*	*Herpes simplex-1*
		Human herpesvirus-2	*Herpes simplex-2*
	Varicellovirus	*Human herpesvirus-3*	*Varicella-zoster virus*
Betaherpesvirinae	*Cytomegalovirus*	*Human herpesvirus-5*	*Human cytomegalovirus*
	Roseolovirus	*Human herpesvirus-6*	
		Human herpesvirus-7	
Gammaherpesvirinae	Lymphocrypto-virus	*Human herpesvirus-4*	*Epstein–Barr virus*

4. TTFFT

Both HSV-1 and HSV-2 are found worldwide. HSV-1 is usually acquired in the first decade of life and spread is enhanced by poor socioeconomic conditions and hygiene. In developed countries about 50–90% of adults have antibody to HSV-1; however in China, for example, it is only 5–10%. Transmission is thought to occur most frequently by oral secretions, presumably kissing. HSV-2 is uncommon before puberty which emphasizes its transmission by genital secretions; in the USA 15–20% of adults have antibody to HSV-2. Transmission of both HSV-1 and HSV-2 occurs more frequently from asymptomatic than symptomatic individuals. Serological studies show that nuns have a very low prevalence of antibody to HSV-2, whereas over 80% of prostitutes have antibody.

5. TTTTT

Herpes simplex viruses can infect any mucocutaneous surface. Herpetic gingivostomatitis is most commonly caused by HSV-1. It is a common childhood infection with painful blisters, fever, malaise and regional lymphadenopathy. It resolves in 2–3 weeks. In adults, primary infection may present as a pharyngitis only. Reactivation later in life results in recurrent herpes labialis which affects one-third of adults in developed countries. These recurrences have been associated with exposure to unusual amounts of sunlight and trauma, among other factors. Frequency of recurrence declines with age. Whitlow is an infection of the digits usually acquired in childhood from stomatitis. In adults it may be a result of genital contact. Encephalitis and keratitis are discussed in Paper 3. Other clinical manifestations of herpes simplex infection are meningitis, tracheobronchitis and proctitis. Disseminated infection may occur in immunocompromised patients. Bell's palsy, transverse myelitis, trigeminal neuralgia and demyelination have also been associated with herpes simplex virus infection.

6. TTTFT

7. TTFTF

The majority of genital tract infections with herpes simplex viruses are asymptomatic. Symptomatic episodes occur either as primary or recurrent infection. Some 'primary' infections are not true primary infections as serology shows previous exposure; these tend to be milder than true primary infections. HSV-2 is the cause of primary genital infection in 50-90% of cases although HSV-1 is becoming more common in some countries. Pre-existing antibody to HSV-1 in a patient with primary infection due to HSV-2 results in a milder illness. In most cases however primary infection due to HSV-1 and HSV-2 cannot be distinguished on clinical grounds. The major difference is that HSV-2 has a 15 times greater recurrence rate than HSV-1. Thus 98% of recurrent genital herpes infections are due to HSV-2. This is in contrast to orolabial herpes where HSV-1 is more likely to recur than HSV-2. After an incubation period of 4-14 days, typical primary attacks begin with a prodromal illness of fever, headache, malaise and myalgia. This is followed by genital soreness, dysuria (and dysparcunia in women). Next, multiple small painful papules appear which develop into vesicles over 24-36 hours. The vesicles become pustular and then form ulcers with surrounding erythema. Over a period of 15-20 days these heal. Regional lymphadenopathy and, in women, cervicitis occur in the majority of cases. Proctitis and pharyngitis are also noted in some cases. In less typical illness where single or large lesions are seen, the differential diagnosis is from primary syphilis (usually painless), chancroid (larger with prominent inguinal lymphadenopathy), trauma, herpes zoster ('cropping' usually seen), drugs (particularly foscarnet), Reiter's disease, Behçet's syndrome, pre-malignant lesions, pyogenic and candidal infections. There are two consequences of primary infection: recurrence and asymptomatic shedding which are not mutually exclusive. Recurrent infections are generally milder and shorter in duration than primary ones. They last a mean of 7–8 days with detectable viral shedding for 3–5 days. Systemic illness is not common and positive cervical cultures are found in only 5% of women. Recurrences also become less frequent over time. Asymptomatic shedding occurs in 0.3–5.4% of infected men and 0.5–8% of infected women at any time. One hospital study has supported the notion that all women post-primary infection shed virus asymptomatically at some time.

8. TTTTF

HSV infection can be transmitted from mother to offspring during the intra-uterine, intra-partum and postnatal periods. *In utero* infection occurs either by transplacental or less commonly by ascending infection. After symptomatic primary genital infection in the mother, spontaneous abortion occurs in up to 25% of women who are 20 weeks pregnant or less. Primary genital infection in the mother between 20 weeks and term is not seemingly associated with such a high risk of fetal mortality but congenital abnormalities may result. These include hydrencephaly, skin scarring, skin vesicles and chorioretinitis. Recurrent infection is far less likely to result in abnormalities. Intra-partum infection accounts for 70–80% of cases of neonatal infection. About one-twentieth to one-third of primary maternal infections at term result in neonatal infection but only 1% of recurrent infections. About 70% of neonatal infection is due to HSV-2. The majority of women with infected offspring do not give a history of previous or current symptomatic infection although viral shedding occurs in 0.09–0.8% of women at term. In the USA 0.03% of deliveries are associated with neonatal HSV. The risk of transmission is increased in the absence of prior maternal antibody, with longer duration of ruptured membranes and the use of fetal scalp monitors.

9. FTTFF

Over 90% of cases of neonatal HSV are symptomatic usually between days 5 and 17 after birth. In 44% of children disease is localized to the skin, eye or mouth. Vesicles are seen in over 80% of these patients by the 11th day. Mortality does not occur but 30% will have neurological sequelae, despite normal CSF findings. Almost all patients will have recurrent skin or mouth lesions. In 56% of cases, encephalitis or disseminated infection occurs. Encephalitis tends to present late (around day 16 or 17) and about one-third will lack skin vesicles. Death occurs in 50% if left untreated, which is reduced to 15% with acyclovir treatment. Over half, whether treated or untreated, will have long-term neurological impairment. This may include psychomotor retardation, microcephaly, blindness, chorioretinitis and learning difficulties. Disseminated disease presents usually on day 4 or 5 with multiple organ derangement, particularly liver, adrenals and CNS. Over 20% will have skin vesicles. If left untreated over 90% will die within the first year of life, this is less than 65% with acyclovir therapy.

10. FFTTT

The prevention of intra-partum transmission is difficult and many measures are tried. One approach has been weekly screening from week 34 of women who give a history of genital herpes possibly combined with routine caesarean section. Both measures are still associated with neonatal HSV. Pre-delivery positive cultures are not necessarily predictive of infection at term and a swab taken at term may not yield a positive culture until after delivery. Caesarean section may not reliably prevent neonatal infection if the membranes have been ruptured for 24 hours or more; it is also unpopular with many women. Moreover, a significant number of women with herpes virus infection do not give a history. The use of prophylactic acyclovir is currently being evaluated. A compromise strategy used in some centres for the mother relies on the following. (1) If a first episode of genital herpes occurs near term, weekly follow-up with vulval and cervical swab cultures are taken until two consecutive cultures are negative. (2) Careful vaginal examination of all women at term. (3) In women with primary infection who are still herpes virus culture-positive near term, caesarean section or acyclovir may be considered. (4) In women with recurrent infection, vaginal delivery is routine unless active lesions are present. (5) Women with active genital herpes are advised to take adequate infection control measures but are not separated from their child. Similarly, breastfeeding is not contraindicated unless there are breast lesions. The use of acyclovir may also reduce the risk of perinatal transmission. Similar measures for the newborn include: (1) babies born to women at 'high-risk' of transmitting infection, particularly those experiencing their first attack in the period 4 weeks before to 4 weeks after birth, are examined daily for signs of infection for the first month of life; (2) routine cultures from eyes, throat and nasopharynx are taken from these babies two to three times per week for the first month; other samples may also be clinically indicated; (3) those babies at high risk of infection should be isolated from other neonates;

and (4) consideration of the uses of immunoprophylaxis or acyclovir prophylaxis. Other family members and visitors with herpes infection, particularly whitlow, may also present a risk to the neonate and contact should be minimized as gloves and masks have not been shown to be reliable.

11. FTTTT

Confirmation of the clinical diagnosis of herpesvirus infection is usually made by culture of the virus from swabs of lesions. Swabs taken from vesicular fluid or from the base of an ulcer are more likely to yield positive cultures than those from dry, erythematous or scabbed lesions. The viruses are thermolabile so if transport of specimens to the laboratory is likely to be more than an hour, specimens should be kept at 4°C in viral transport medium. The virus will grow in commonly used cell lines within 24–48 hours. Other tests such as electron microscopy of vesicular fluid and serology are used occasionally. PCR is finding a role in the diagnosis of herpes encephalitis. Differentiation between HSV-1 and HSV-2 may help as a prognostic marker in neonatal and genital herpes infections. This is most commonly done by the use of specific monoclonal antibodies in an immunofluorescence test of cultured virus. Other tests employed are: growth on chick allantoic membranes (HSV-1 produces pocks smaller than 0.75 mm diameter, HSV-2 greater than 1 mm); culture in unusual cell lines where the cytopathic effects can be differentiated; restriction enzyme digestion of viral DNA; antibody-based techniques such as ELISA or neutralization.

12. FTTTT

Antiviral drugs that are effective against herpes simplex viruses are acyclovir, phosphonoformate, idoxuridine and vidarabine. Acyclovir is now the drug of choice for almost all indications. Oral acyclovir prophylaxis has been found to reduce the frequency of recurrence of genital herpes and is used in patients with six or more recurrences per year. It has been given for many years without significant adverse effect. Some physicians also recommend acyclovir prophylaxis for patients (in particular those that are immunocompromised) with frequently recurring oral herpes. In patients with less than six attacks per year, topical 5% acyclovir has been shown to reduce the duration of symptoms but the cost-benefit aspect would not make this a firm recommendation. An ointment containing surfactants has been used successfully in the past but has been superseded by acyclovir. Disseminated infections and encephalitis should be treated with intravenous acyclovir at least initially.

MOLLUSCUM CONTAGIOSUM

13. TFTTT
Molluscum contagiosum is a poxvirus. On the basis of genome analysis, two subtypes are recognized. Type 1 is responsible for over 90% of all infections. Unlike the herpes simplex virus the two molluscum contagiosum subtypes do not exhibit anatomic preference. The virus is transmitted by direct skin-to-skin contact particularly in moist environments such as swimming pools. It is common in children worldwide. It is estimated that 1% of all populations in developed countries will experience molluscum contagiosum. Sexual transmission has increased in some countries.

14. TTTFF
Whether genital or elsewhere, there are typically 2-20 lesions which appear after an incubation period of 15–40 days. These are characteristically painless pearly-white nodules, 2–5 mm in diameter, with central umbilication. A cheesy material can be expressed from their core. Uncommonly, large single lesions may be seen, or they are pruritic. Lesions affecting the eyelid are often accompanied by conjunctivitis. Spontaneous resolution occurs in about 2 months. The diagnosis is clinical but can be supported by electron microscopic examination of exudate for virus. Treatment is for cosmetic reasons and can be by cryotherapy, electrodesiccation or local chemicals (phenol, silver nitrate, trichloroacetic acid). Cantharidin has been used successfully on non-genital lesions but is irritant. Podophyllin is ineffective and laser treatment is associated with scarring.

HUMAN PAPILLOMAVIRUSES

15. FFFTT
*Papillomaviruses are historically classified on the basis of morphology with the polyomaviruses in the family **Papovaviridae**. Biologically and genetically these are very different group of viruses and do not share antigenic structure. Papillomaviruses are non-enveloped viruses with icosahedral capsids of 52–55 nm in diameter; polyomaviruses are smaller at 38–43 nm diameter. The viruses are poorly immunogenic and do not grow reliably in cell culture. They are subclassified on the basis of genomic differences into over 60 types. All the viruses have tropism for epithelial cells but different types have a predilection for specific tissue, e.g. the common types associated with the genital tract, human*

papillomaviruses (HPV) 6 and 11, are rarely found elsewhere on the
body. They can persist in infected cells either as free DNA (the genome
is a circle of double-stranded DNA) or become integrated into host DNA.
In the latter process the virus loses some of its genes.

16. TTTFF

Human papillomavirus (HPV) infections are ubiquitous worldwide.
Non-genital warts occur most frequently in children and early adolescence:
5–10% of schoolchildren will have cutaneous warts in the USA. It is
estimated that over 90% of infections are subclinical. Transmission of
HPV is predominantly by direct contact but fomite transmission has also
been recorded especially with activities such as gymnastics and
swimming. Virus can also be detected in the undergarments of 20%
of people with genital warts although transmission by clothing would
be an unusual route. HPV is moderately infectious; about 60% of sexual
contacts of individuals with genital warts will acquire infection.

17. TTFTT

Table 7.4 shows the clinical associations of human papillomaviruses.
Verruca vulgaris or common warts are sessile and usually multiple.
Verruca plantaris are usually single, flat warts on the feet. A hand version
is known as Butcher's warts. Juvenile warts, also flat, tend to occur
on the face and the extremities. As the name suggests, these occur mainly
in children. Oral papillomas are the commonest benign epithelial tumours
of the mouth and are usually pedunculated and single. Unlike lesions
at other sites, they rarely recur after being excised. Focal epithelial
hyperplasia (Heck's tumour) presents as flat or slightly elevated plaques
in the mouth. They are usually multiple and appear mainly in certain
races, such as the Eskimo Indians. Laryngeal papillomas are the
commonest benign tumours of the larynx. They are thought to arise by
perinatal transmission from the birth canal. They usually present with
hoarseness or dysphonia and rarely as respiratory distress. The disease
has a bimodal distribution, at first in children under 5 years of age and
then in young adults. Spontaneous resolution often occurs at puberty
in the former group. Malignant transformation has occurred after
radiation therapy. Management is surgical although interferon therapy
has also been used. Epidermodysplasia verruciformis is a rare, autosomal
recessive disease which results in defective cell-mediated immunity. The
patients are unusually susceptible to cutaneous HPV infection and 25%
will develop squamous carcinoma of the skin. HPV-5 and HPV-8 appear
to be associated with skin malignancy. HPV-5 also causes warts in
patients with other forms of poor cell-mediated immunity, such as

post-renal transplantation, and may cause squamous cell carcinoma in these patients. HPV-11 has been a rare cause of conjunctival papilloma.

Table 7.4 Disease manifestations of human papillomaviruses

Disease		Common HPV types	Less common HPV types
Cutaneous	Common warts	2, 26, 28, 29	1, 4, 49
	Plantar warts	1, 4	
	Flat warts	3, 10, 27	46
	Butcher's warts	7	
	Epidermodysplasia verruciformis	3, 5, 8, 9, 10, 12, 14, 15, 17, 19, 20–25, 36, 46–50	
	Squamous cell carcinoma	5, 8	41, 48, 55
	Malignant melanoma		38 (rare)
	Conjunctival papilloma	11	
Oral	Oral papilloma	Various	
	Heck's tumour	13, 32	
	Multiple papillomatosis	6, 11	57
	Keratoacanthoma		37
Respiratory tract	Laryngeal papillomatosis	11, 16	6
	Laryngeal carcinoma	16, 18	30, 6, 11
Genital tract	Condyloma acuminata	6, 11	10, 31, others
	Cervical intra-epithelial neoplasia	16, 18	3, 6, 11, 31, 33, 35, 42–45, 51, 52, 56, 57
	Vulval intra-epithelial neoplasia	6, 11, 16	42
	Genital malignancy	16, 18, 33	51, 54
	Bowenoid papulosis	16, 18	

18. TTTTT

Human papillomaviruses are classically associated with condyloma acuminata, obvious wart-like lesions. These need to be differentiated from condyloma lata of secondary syphilis. The majority of such lesions (about 65%) are caused by HPV-6, with 20% due to HPV-11. Occasionally condyloma become very large and are known as Buschke–Lowenstein tumours; these are typically benign and rarely metastasize. Apart from the verrucous type, flat condyloma are not uncommon. Approximately 10% of women with vulval warts will also have obvious cervical warts but over 50% will have microscopic evidence of cervical HPV infection. In men only 5% of patients with external warts will have urethral involvement. Warts tend to be larger and more extensive during pregnancy but regress spontaneously after delivery. More prevalent than cervical condyloma are cytological abnormalities of the cervix, so-called cervical intra-epithelial neoplasia (CIN). Identical abnormalities of the anus (AIN), vulva (VIN), vagina (VaIN) and penis (PIN) have also been described. CIN is the best studied and is of three histological grades. (1) CIN-1: mild dysplasia, 85% of these will regress. (2) Moderate dysplasia. (3) Severe dysplasia and carcinoma *in situ*. HPV can be detected in practically all CIN lesions. Epidemiologically the majority of low-grade lesions are associated with HPV-6 or HPV-11. The majority of high-grade lesions are associated with HPV-16. Bowenoid papulosis is a pre-malignant condition that occurs on the external genitalia of both sexes. It often regresses. Recent studies have shown that HPV, in particular HPV-16, can be found in the majority of genital cancers. HPV is likely to be a major but not the sole factor in the genesis of these cancers. Acetowhite lesions are areas of whitening which appear after staining with 5% aqueous acetic acid. There is good (but not absolute) correlation with the presence of HPV in the stained cells.

19. TTTFT
Cervical cancer and other genital malignancies have been thought for some decades to be of infective aetiology. HPV is the prime culprit in the light of current evidence. (1) Epidemiological: HPV is almost always found in the tumours. (2) Animal studies: bovine and rabbit papilloma-viruses cause malignancies in their respective hosts. (3) Human studies: patients with epidermodysplasia verruciformis develop squamous carcinoma of the skin after HPV infection and long-term exposure to sunlight. (4) Laboratory: papillomaviruses contain genes that can transform cells *in vitro*. It is quite clear, however, that cofactors must be involved. (1) Other infections: herpes simplex virus infection is a strong risk factor. (2) Smoking: products of smoking have been shown to cause DNA aberrations in cervical cells. Smoking *per se* is also a strong risk factor. (3) Hormonal factors: prolonged use of oral contra-ceptives is epidemiologically associated with high risk. There is also laboratory evidence that oestrogens can induce malignant change in HPV-infected cells. (4) Immunosuppression. (5) Vitamin A deficiency. Irradiation, chronic exposure to sunlight and trauma have been implicated as cofactors in the genesis of HPV-induced squamous cell carcinoma at other sites but not of the genital tract.

20. TFTTF
Typical wart lesions do not pose much diagnostic difficulty. It is the less obvious infection for which laboratory investigations have a role. As the effect of HPV infection, rather than the mere presence of virus,

is medically important, tests used to detect cytological abnormalities are mainly used. (1) Acetowhite staining: application of 5% acetic acid facilitates the detection of subepithelial lesions. Acetic acid coagulates epidermal proteins and leads to white plaques which when magnified by colposcopy reveal 'micro-warts'. There is a good correlation with HPV infection although there is a high false-negative rate if magnification is not used. (2) Cytology: cytological examination of smears is used as a screening method. One particular finding, koilocytosis (marked perinuclear vacuolation), is almost pathognomonic of HPV infection. (3) Histology: gives more detailed information than cytology.

More specific diagnosis of HPV infection depends on gene detection methods as the virus cannot be cultivated *in vitro* and is a poor inducer of antibodies. Two methods, Southern blotting and PCR, are widely used.

21. TTTTT
Specific antiviral agents against HPV are not yet available and most commonly used remedies are directed at removing the epithelial excess induced by the virus. The majority of cutaneous warts will spontaneously regress over a period of weeks to months. Treatment for cosmetic reasons is often successful with topical salicylate paste, formalin or glutaraldehyde. Other physical methods are used in hospitals: excision, cryotherapy or laser treatment. Genital warts are routinely treated with the repeated topical application of the cytotoxic agents, podophyllin and podophyllotoxin, at concentrations of 10–25%. Podophyllotoxin is an active constituent of podophyllin and is less toxic. There is also a lower risk of mutagenicity with prolonged use. Agents that have been used in specialist centres include 5-fluorouracil (a cytotoxic agent used for the treatment of some cancers), topical trichloroacetic acid and intralesional alpha-interferon. Idoxuridine has been shown to be ineffective. The recurrence rate is high whatever the treatment. Efforts are being made to develop a vaccine but none is yet available.

Paper 8   Retroviruses and AIDS

INTRODUCTION

1. TFFTT

One of the central tenets of molecular biology can be summarized as 'DNA makes RNA makes protein'. This maxim stipulates the direction of flow of genetic information. However retroviruses possess the ability to manufacture a DNA copy of their RNA genome by virtue of the enzyme reverse transcriptase. This apparent 'backward' step led to the adoption of the term 'retroviruses' to describe this family of viruses. Retroviruses are widespread throughout nature. In fact the human retroviruses are among the most recent to be discovered. Retroviruses thus possess RNA genomes in the form of two identical copies of single-stranded RNA. They are enveloped, the envelope being acquired as mature virions bud through host cell membranes. Possession of an envelope makes these viruses fairly fragile as loss of the envelope results in loss of infectivity. Retroviruses are divided taxonomically into three subfamilies, the **Oncovirinae, Lentivirinae** *and* **Spumavirinae.** *The* **Oncovirinae** *are further subdivided on the basis of virion morphology into B-, C- and D-type viruses. Most are C-type, the characteristic feature of which is that no intracytoplasmic viral structures can be observed until the virus begins budding at the cell membrane. Endogenous genetic elements with retrovirus-like sequences are classified as C-type oncoviruses. All retroviruses carry at least three genes in the order 5'-gag-pol-env-3',* gag *encoding internal structural proteins,* pol *encoding the reverse transcriptase and* env *the envelope proteins. Many oncogenic retroviruses carry in addition cellular genes which may cause neoplastic transformation and are therefore known as oncogenes.*

HUMAN RETROVIRUSES

2. FTTFF

The only well-characterized retroviruses of humans identified thus far are human T cell lymphotropic virus types 1 and 2 (HTLV-1 and HTLV-II), human immunodeficiency virus types 1 and 2 (HIV-1 and HIV-2) and human foamy virus. These belong to the onco-, lenti- and spumavirus genera, respectively. The relationship of human foamy virus to disease remains unclear although there has been recent interest in the role of this virus in the pathogenesis of autoimmune thyroid disease. In addition, expression of non-infectious endogenous C-type oncoviruses has been detected in the placenta and in some teratocarcinomas. Human B cell lymphotropic virus (HBLV) was the name initially given to the virus now known as human herpesvirus type 6 and is therefore a herpesvirus. JC and BK viruses, named after the initials of the patients from whom they were isolated, are papovaviruses. SIV stands for Simian immunodeficiency virus. This is a retrovirus but not of humans. SIV infection of certain monkeys causes a simian immunodeficiency syndrome similar to AIDS (known as SAIDS) and thus provides an excellent model for the investigation of the pathogenesis of AIDS and for the testing of putative antiviral agents and vaccines.

HUMAN T CELL LYMPHOTROPIC VIRUSES

3. FFTTF
Epidemiological studies of HTLV-I infection have identified a number of highly endemic pockets restricted to four geographic regions in the world: Japan, where there are over one million carriers; the Caribbean islands, predominantly in citizens of African descent; Central and South America, particularly in Panama and Columbia; and equatorial Africa, although here the epidemiology is less clear. HTLV-I was first isolated from the leukaemic cells of a patient with adult T cell leukaemia/ lymphoma (ATLL) and further studies have confirmed an aetiological link between HTLV-I and ATLL. HTLV-II was first isolated from hairy cell leukaemia cells although the pathogenic role of HTLV-II in that disease is unclear. HTLV-I is also associated with inflammatory and degenerative diseases of the central and peripheral nervous system and skeletal muscles. The CNS diseases referred to as HTLV-I associated myelopathy (HAM) in Japan and tropical spastic paraparesis (TSP) in the Caribbean, are clinically identical syndromes (8.6). There have been suggestions that HTLV-I may be associated with polymyositis in Japan and the Caribbean. HTLV-I (and HTLV-II) infection frequently occurs as a co-infection with HIV, primarily in intravenous drug abusers. Such co-infection has been associated with the accelerated progression of AIDS. HTLV-I does infect CD4-positive T lymphocytes but the CD4 molecule itself is not the cellular receptor for the virus.

4. TTTFT
HTLV-I is a cell-associated virus and thus efficient transmission of the virus requires transfer of infected cells. Worldwide the two most

common modes of transmission are vertical and sexual. The exact mode of vertical spread is believed to be via breast milk rather than transplacentally or perinatally. Studies of bottle-feeding in Japan have demonstrated a decreased incidence of infection in the offspring of infected mothers. Blood transfusion is a very efficient means of spread although the potential for transmission declines with storage of the blood products. Sharing of needles among injectable drug users also transmits infection. In contrast to HIV, haemophiliacs are not a high-risk group for HTLV-I infection. This reflects the acellular nature of the blood products administered to these patients.

ADULT T CELL LEUKAEMIA

5. TFTTF

ATLL may have several clinical presentations from an acute leukaemia to a predominantly cutaneous lymphoma. Whatever the initial presentation, it most commonly culminates as a highly malignant monoclonal proliferation of CD4-positive T cells which express large amounts of the receptor for interleukin-2. As with other virus-associated malignancies, there is a long latent period (e.g. 30–40 years) from seroconversion to development of disease. The lifetime risk of ATLL for seropositive patients is estimated to be 2% in Japanese patients infected at birth or 4% in Jamaicans infected before the age of 20 years. The presence of the HTLV-I genome, in proviral (DNA) form, integrated into the leukaemic cell chromosomal DNA is clearly demonstrable by Southern blotting. Hypercalcaemia is a common feature of the disease and may result from release of cytokines with osteoclast activating properties. Hypocalcaemia has also been reported late in the illness. The first-line therapy of this monoclonal malignancy is aggressive chemotherapy. Antiviral agents such as AZT have not been shown to be of much use.

TROPICAL PARAPARESIS/HTLV-I ASSOCIATED MYELOPATHY (TSP/HAM)

6. FFFTF

The mean age of onset of TSP is about 40 years. Most studies report a female : male preponderance of 2 : 1. Presentation is usually insidious with chronic progression of stiffness or weakness in one or both legs resulting in spastic paraparesis. Urinary frequency, urgency and penile impotence are common. Although many patients describe various symptoms, such as numbness and burning, only minor sensory signs are elicited on formal examination. Ten years after contracting the disease, 30% of patients are bedridden and 45% cannot walk unaided by crutches. Cranial nerves are usually spared. The lifetime incidence of TSP in HTLV-I-infected individuals is approximately 0.25%. TSP/HAM has been described wherever pockets of HTLV-I infection have been found. Incidence is high in HTLV-I endemic areas. In the UK, TSP has been described in several individuals, mostly of Afro-Caribbean origin. Antibodies to HTLV-I are found in the serum and CSF of patients with TSP, often at very high titre. Only moderate numbers of white cells ($<50 \times 10^6/l$) are found in the CSF. ATLL-like cells may be found in the CSF at very low frequency. HTLV-1 DNA is readily demonstrable in peripheral blood cells. To date, no major differences between 'leukaemogenic' and 'neurogenic' strains of HTLV-1 have been reported. Many forms of therapy have been tried in TSP/HAM. Steroids may be of short-term benefit but long-term follow-up shows no difference in outcome between treated and non-treated patients.

HUMAN T LYMPHOTROPIC VIRUS-II

7. FTTTF

HTLV-I and HTLV-II are similar in structure with extensive regions of partial nucleic acid homology. Both viruses infect CD4-positive T lymphocytes. HTLV-II was originally considered an innocuous virus. It is now thought to play a pathogenic role in a number of diseases. Cases of HTLV-II neurological disease similar to HAM and characterized by slowly progressive leg weakness, spasticity and bladder and bowel dysfunction have been identified. Large granulocytic cell leukaemia has been reported in patients with antibodies to HTLV-II. Several cases of cutaneous diseases ranging from eczema to debilitating lymphocytic infiltration of the skin have also been described in association with HTLV-II infection. Diagnosis is by detection of antibodies to the virus. However, between 10% and 40% of HTLV-II infected persons are negative when tested in current HTLV-I antibody assays. Thus screening of the blood supply for HTLV-I infected donors, as occurs in the USA and Australia, will not pick up all HTLV-II carriers. Clusters of HTLV-II seropositive intravenous drug abusers have been observed in London and the USA. The incidence of HTLV-II in drug users is much higher than that of HTLV-I.

HUMAN IMMUNODEFICIENCY VIRUSES

8. TTFFT
The molecular biology of HIV is known in enormous detail. The 9 kb RNA genome of HIV contains gag-, *pol- and* env- *genes, as do all retroviruses. However, HIV has at least six other additional genes (*vif, vpu, vpr, tat, rev *and* nef*), the products of which appear to regulate the rate of replication of genome. The* gag *gene encodes four nucleocapsid proteins (p24, p17, p9 and p7), each of which is proteolytically cleaved from a 53 kDa* gag *precursor by the HIV protease. The* pol *gene contains the reverse transcriptase, DNA integrase, and protease proteins, all of which are potential targets for antiviral drugs. The* env *gene encodes the gp160 precursor glycoprotein which is broken down to form the gp120 and gp41 proteins in the mature virion. The glycosylation of these proteins is performed by host cell enzymes.*

9. FTFFF
HIV specifically infects CD4+ T lymphocytes and monocytes because this transmembrane antigen on each of these cells represents the principal high-affinity cellular receptor for this virus. HIV may also infect other cell types, e.g. glial cells, gut epithelium and bone marrow progenitors. Whether infection of these cells is mediated via receptors other than CD4 is an active area of investigation. Certain strains of HIV preferentially infect monocytes and macrophages whereas others display selectivity for T cells. Amino acid differences in the env *gene may underlie these tropic distinctions. Having gained access to a cell, the viral genome is uncoated and reverse transcription occurs. Reverse transcriptase is not an accurate enzyme: a number of base changes may be incorporated by mistake into the DNA version of the virus. This infidelity underlies the rapid rate of emergence of viral mutants within an infected host. The double-stranded DNA provirus is incorporated into host cell chromosomal DNA via the action of the viral DNA integrase enzyme. The virus is able to remain in a latent state once this has been achieved. HIV does not replicate within resting T cells, presumably because critical host factors are absent. Activation of T cells* in vitro, *by any of several methods, enables a high level of HIV replication to occur.*

TRANSMISSION OF HIV

10. TTTFF
HIV is spread by sexual contact, exposure to infected blood or blood products and vertical transmission from mother to child. While

intercourse between men may be more efficient at transmitting virus than that between men and women, heterosexual spread does occur. Transmission via this route is enhanced by the presence of genital ulceration, whatever the cause, and is more likely to occur from male to female than female to male. Large numbers of haemophiliacs acquired HIV infection in the early days of the epidemic through factor VIII pools. However, blood products can be rendered safe by heat treatment. The virus is present in breast milk and there are documented cases of children becoming HIV-infected by breastfeeding from mothers who themselves acquired HIV infection post-natally from blood transfusion. There is no evidence to suggest that HIV may be transmitted by droplet spread. Although a theoretical possibility, there are no data to suggest that insect-borne spread occurs.

11. TFFTF

Knowledge of this aspect of HIV biology is accumulating through the establishment of large multi-centre collaborative surveys. The European Collaborative Study has published data relating to over 700 pregnancies involving HIV-positive mothers. Vertical transmission was associated with maternal p24 antigenaemia and a CD4 count of less than $700/\mu l$. The transmission rate therefore varies according to the status of the maternal population under study. The overall rate in the European study was around 15% and similar figures have been reported from other studies. The diagnosis of HIV infection in the neonate is complicated by the passage of maternal antibodies across the placenta. Thus the presence of anti-HIV antibody at or near birth in the neonate is not evidence of infection. Serological diagnosis of infection can only be made routinely by demonstrating the persistence of anti-HIV beyond 18 months of age. The mode of infection of the offspring is unclear. There is evidence to suggest that viral transmission can occur transplacentally, perinatally and postnatally via breast milk. The relative importance of these three routes is the subject of current investigation. Although the majority of infected children will have shown some feature of HIV infection by 12 months of age, the mortality rate in the European study was of the order of 20% with a further 10% having AIDS.

12. FFFTT

Large-scale prospective surveys (of over 2600 incidents) have estimated that the overall HIV transmission rate after inoculation of infected blood via an occupational percutaneous injury is 0.3%. Similar studies have failed to document a single case of transmission following splashing of HIV-infected material onto intact skin. There are case reports of transmission following splashing of mucous membranes with HIV-infected material but the risk is likely to be considerably smaller than that for percutaneous injury. Despite initial high hopes, there are now a number of reports of failed AZT prophylaxis given following a known exposure incident, even when the AZT has been initiated within 1 hour of exposure. It will be statistically impossible to demonstrate whether AZT prophylaxis may nevertheless be of some benefit in reducing transmission. HIV, being an envelope virus, is relatively fragile and easily inactivated. However, the virus may survive if present in a protein-rich environment such as dried blood and experiments on recovery of virus have demonstrated survival for up to 7 days. Any agent which destroys the lipid envelope of HIV will render the virus non-infectious.

LABORATORY DIAGNOSIS OF HIV INFECTION

13. FFTFT
The mainstay of routine laboratory diagnosis of HIV infection is the demonstration of specific antibodies to the virus in serum (or saliva) from the patient. Thus the presence of anti-HIV antibody is accepted as definitive evidence of infection. However, anti-HIV antibody will not be present as soon as the patient becomes infected with the virus. The period between infection and the generation of detectable anti-HIV is termed the 'window period'. During this period, an individual is infected with HIV but is anti-HIV antibody-negative. In the majority of patients this period is of the order of 3 months. Various attempts have been made to devise alternative diagnostic approaches to avoid the problems created by the window period. None has so far been reliable enough to have been adopted into routine practice. The p24 antigen test may be positive during the window period but prospective studies have shown that the sensitivity of this test is well below 100%, so a negative p24 test is difficult to interpret. Culture of HIV requires specialized expertise and facilities. In any case, during the phase of asymptomatic carriage of HIV, it may not be possible to isolate virus from peripheral blood. Culture is therefore not a reasonable approach to diagnosis. The consequences of a diagnosis of HIV infection are of such significance that it is accepted medical practice not to perform HIV diagnostic assays without patient consent, other than in exceptional circumstances (e.g. when the patient is unable to give consent). In addition, it is good practice not to accept an anti-HIV antibody-positive result on a single serum sample but to insist that the result be confirmed by testing a second sample from the same patient.

ACUTE HIV INFECTION

14. TTFFF

An acute mononucleosis-like syndrome occurs 1–6 weeks after exposure to HIV in about one-half to two-thirds of patients. The CDC classification system (Table 8.1) lists this retroviral syndrome as category 1 of HIV disease. This period is associated with high levels of viraemia and HIV is widely disseminated during this early stage of infection. Patients with this syndrome are therefore infectious. HIV antibodies are usually detectable by ELISA after 2–3 months. There are no data to suggest that the long-term prognosis in these patients is any different from those who undergo an asymptomatic seroconversion.

Table 8.1 CDC classification system of HIV infection

Group I. Acute infection

Group II. Asymptomatic infection

Group III. Persistent generalized lymphadenopathy.

Group IV. Other diseases
    Subgroup A. Constitutional disease
    Subgroup B. Neurological disease
    Subgroup C. Secondary infectious diseases
        Category C-1. Specified secondary infectious diseases listed in the CDC surveillance definition for AIDS (Table 8.2)
        Category C-2. Other specified secondary infectious diseases
    Subgroup D. Secondary malignancies
    Subgroup E. Other conditions

ACQUIRED IMMUNODEFICIENCY SYNDROME (AIDS)

15. FTFFT

HIV infection is a necessary but not sufficient cause of AIDS. In other words, HIV-infected individuals may exhibit a range of clinical consequences from asymptomatic infection through to the severe debilitating immunodeficiency state known as AIDS. The mean incubation period from HIV infection to the manifestation of AIDS is now of the order of 7–10 years. Little is known of cofactors which may influence the development of AIDS in HIV-positive individuals: co-infections such as concurrent human herpesvirus 6, cytomegalovirus, HTLV-I and *Mycoplasma*, as well as environmental factors, have been implicated. The CDC Surveillance Case Definition for AIDS (Table 8.2) has been widely adopted to assist in the diagnosis of AIDS in an individual patient. *Pneumocystis carinii* pneumonia

Table 8.2 AIDS-defining illnesses (adapted from CDC Surveillance Case Definition for AIDS 1992)

(i) Patients with no other cause of immunodeficiency but without confirmation of HIV infection:
Systemic candidiasis
Extrapulmonary cryptococcosis
Cryptosporidiosis >1 month
CMV infection of any organ other than liver, spleen or lymph nodes in patients
  > 1 month old
Prolonged mucocutaneous HSV infection, HSV pneumonitis or oesophagitis
Kaposi's sarcoma in patients <60 years old
Primary CNS lymphoma in patients <60 years old
Lymphoid interstitial pneumonitis in patients <13 years old
Mycobacterium avium complex or disseminated *M. kansasii*
Pneumocystis carinii pneumonia
Progressive multifocal leucoencephalopathy
Cerebral toxoplasmosis in patients >1 month old

(ii) Known HIV-infected patients
Recurrent pyogenic bacterial infections in patients >13 years old
Disseminated coccidioidomycosis
Disseminated histoplasmosis
Isosporiasis >1 month duration
Kaposi's sarcoma at any age
Primary CNS lymphoma at any age
Non-Hodgkin's lymphoma
Disseminated mycobacterial disease, other than *M. tuberculosis*
Extrapulmonary tuberculosis
Recurrent *Salmonella* septicaemia
Oesophageal candidiasis[a]
CMV retinitis[a]
Lymphoid interstitial pneumonitis in patients <13 years old[a]
Pneumocystis carinii pneumonia[a]
Cerebral toxoplasmosis in patients >1 month old[a]
HIV encephalopathy[a]
HIV wasting syndrome[a]

[a] Diseases diagnosed presumptively

(PCP) is the commonest AIDS-defining illness. Herpes zoster, oral candidiasis and oral hairy leukoplakia are all considerably more common in HIV-infected individuals than in age- and sex-matched controls. While the occurrence of any of these manifestations, which reflect an underlying immunodeficiency, may herald the imminent onset of AIDS, they do not of themselves constitute AIDS-defining illnesses. Persistent generalized lymphadenopathy (PGL) is another common clinical feature of HIV infection but prospective studies have shown that PGL is not associated with an increased risk of developing AIDS than is asymptomatic infection without lymphadenopathy. The case definition for AIDS may well be altered as the list of diseases recognized as complications of HIV infection increases. A recent modification to include the presence of a CD4 cell count of less than 200, carcinoma of the uterine cervix in women and tuberculosis as AIDS-defining illnesses has recently been adopted in the USA. These modifications have not, for various reasons, found universal acceptance in Europe.

16. TTTTT

The exact mechanisms whereby HIV infection leads to such profound immunodeficiency are not clear. A large number of possible mechanisms have been proposed and there is extensive evidence to support the existence of many of these. Thus, HIV infection of CD4 cells in vitro *is usually cytolytic. HIV-infected individuals do possess cytotoxic T cells (CTL) capable of destroying HIV-infected target cells. The development of these cells may be important in overcoming HIV replication and spread in the early stages of infection. However, the magnitude of the loss of CD4 cells in AIDS cannot be accounted for by loss of HIV-infected cells only. Thus, virus-induced autoimmune attack on uninfected CD4 cells, and the excess production of gp120 from infected cells binding to uninfected cells and thereby rendering those cells as targets for CTL and ADCC activity, have been suggested as ways in which uninfected cells may be destroyed. Many of the functions of macrophages and monocytes, including antigen presentation are impaired by HIV infection. The role of the lymphoid organs in the pathogenesis of HIV infection has been the subject of much recent interest. Although most studies have necessarily concentrated on HIV infection of peripheral blood cells, it is becoming clear that this has led to a misleading picture. Viral burden detectable in lymph nodes is considerably higher than in peripheral blood and the lymphoid organs may function as reservoirs of HIV infection, actively trapping circulating free virus and virus-infected cells. The follicular dendritic cells are pivotal in this activity. As the network of follicular dendritic cells degenerates as a result of HIV infection, the ability of lymphoid organs to trap HIV particles declines. This coincides with the reappearance of viraemia and the emergence of AIDS.*

17. TTFTT

The clinical manifestations of AIDS are protean. For epidemiological and comparative purposes, they are broadly categorized into neurological,

Table 8.3 Common clinical manifestations in AIDS

System	Presentation	Causative organism disease
Pulmonary	Pneumonia	*Pneumocystis carinii*
		Mycobacterium tuberculosis
		Cytomegalovirus
		Cryptococcus neoformans
		Aspergillosis
		Histoplasmosis
	Tumour	Lymphoma
		Kaposi's sarcoma
Gastrointestinal	Candidiasis	*Candida albicans*
	Oral hairy leukoplakia	Epstein–Barr virus
	Oral ulcers	Herpes simplex virus
		Cytomegalovirus
	Oesophagitis	Herpes simplex virus
		Cytomegalovirus
	Colitis	Cytomegalovirus
	Diarrhoea	*Salmonella* species
		Shigella species
		Giardia lamblia
		Cryptosporidium species
		Isospora bellii
		Entamoeba histolytica
Central nervous system	Brain abscess	*Toxoplasma gondii*
	Aseptic meningitis	Part of seroconverting illness – may be HIV-related
	Meningitis	*Cryptococcus neoformans*
	Encephalitis	Cytomegalovirus, HIV, *M. tuberculosis*
	Retinitis	Cytomegalovirus
	Progressive multifocal leucoencephalopathy	JC and BK virus
	Tumour	Kaposi's sarcoma
		Primary lymphoma
		Metastatic lymphoma
Skin	Ulcers	Herpes simplex
	Shingles	Varicella-zoster
	Multiple nodules	*Cryptococcus neoformans*
Reticuloendothelial	Lymphadenopathy	*Toxoplasma gondii*
		M. avium-intracellulare
		Epstein–Barr virus
Malignancy		Kaposi's sarcoma
		Non-Hodgkin's lymphoma
		Burkitt's lymphoma
		Lymphoproliferative disease
		Hodgkin's lymphoma
		Squamous carcinoma
		Testicular tumours
		Basal cell carcinoma
		Melanoma
		Carcinoma of uterine cervix

infectious and malignant complications. A list of common manifestations is given in Table 8.3. The relative frequency of these will vary in different patient groups. The spectrum of opportunistic infections, particularly, will reflect the pattern of infectious organisms extant in a given geographical location.

18. FFFTT

PCP infection commonly occurs in early life without resulting in clinical disease. Immunosuppression from whatever cause can lead to reactivation of this infection, resulting in a life-threatening intra-alveolar pneumonitis. Diagnosis is by demonstration of *P. carinii* cysts in clinical material. The cysts can be identified by special staining reactions (e.g. with silver) or by immunofluorescence using monoclonal antibodies. However, spontaneously produced sputum is not necessarily an adequate sample for diagnosis: the cysts may not be coughed up from their location deep in the lower respiratory tract. Either an induced sputum sample (obtained following inhalation of nebulized saline) or bronchoalveolar lavage fluid obtained at bronchoscopy is necessary for accurate diagnosis. Toxoplasmosis is the commonest cause of intracranial mass lesions in AIDS patients. However, definitive diagnosis is difficult. The diagnosis is strongly suggested by the presence of multiple ring-enhancing lesions on CT scan. However, many toxoplasmic abscesses are not detected by CT scanning and a pragmatic approach to diagnosis is to determine whether the lesions respond to an empirical course of therapy for toxoplasmosis. Measurement of antibody responses to *Toxoplasma* is of little diagnostic value. *Cryptococcus neoformans* is a fungus and therefore cannot be identified by Gram-staining. The organism is present in the CSF during cryptococcal meningitis and can be seen by India ink staining. However, a more reliable approach is to isolate the organism or demonstrate the presence of cryptococcal antigen by an appropriate immunological methodology. Measurement of the titre of antigen may be useful in monitoring response to treatment and the emergence of relapsing disease. *Mycobacterium avium-intracellulare* complex (MAC) disease presents most commonly with fevers, night sweats, fatigue and weight loss. Multiple organs may be infected but hepatosplenomegaly and diffuse lymphadenopathy are the commonest clinical findings. Patients have a continuous bacteraemia and thus infection can be diagnosed by culture of the blood on appropriate growth medium. The immunosuppression in AIDS is not reversible and even though patients may recover from the acute opportunistic infections which they may suffer, all of these infections have a propensity to recur. The emphasis in managing HIV-infected patients is therefore directed towards prevention of opportunist infections by appropriate prophylactic therapy. This may result in HIV-positive patients being on a considerable cocktail of antimicrobial agents.

HUMAN IMMUNODEFICIENCY VIRUS-2 (HIV-2)

19. TTFFF

HIV-2 was isolated from West African patients with AIDS in 1986. The new virus undoubtedly belonged to the HIV group but differed significantly from HIV-1. There is evidence to suggest that HIV-2 has been present in West Africa since at least 1966. In many West African countries, it is the prevalent HIV strain with HIV-1 infection being rare. Analysis of the nucleotide sequence of isolates of HIV-2 shows only around 40% similarity to HIV-1 but 75% similarity to certain strains of SIV, particularly SIV_{SM} (SIV from West African sooty mangabey monkeys). The shared geographic distribution of HIV-2 and SIV_{SM}, together with the genomic similarities between the two viruses, offers the strongest evidence to date that HIVs may have been transmitted from monkeys to humans. Only about 80% of sera from HIV-2 infected individuals cross-react in HIV-1 antibody ELISAs. Anti-HIV-1 antibody testing alone will therefore not identify all HIV-2 infected donors. Screening of the blood supply for both HIV-1 and HIV-2 was introduced in the UK in 1992. A number of HIV-2 infected individuals have been identified in the UK. Nearly all of these give a history of some connection with West Africa. Although both HIV-1 and HIV-2 infection can lead to AIDS, the rate of progression of disease is some ten times greater for HIV-1. Individuals with HIV-2 infection are therefore less likely to develop AIDS or, at least, will have a much longer asymptomatic period.

AIDS THERAPY

20. FTTTF

Zidovudine (azidothymidine, AZT) was the first reverse transcriptase inhibitor to be licensed. Following the success of this drug in early trials a number of structural analogues were assessed in the search for greater selectivity of action. Two of these have now been approved for use in the treatment of HIV infection by the US Food and Drug Administration: Zalcitabine (dideoxycytidine, ddC) and Didanosine (dideoxyinosine, ddI). All of these drugs are known as dideoxynucleosides because they lack hydroxyl groups on the 2' and 3' positions of the sugar ring. Once phosphorylated these drugs inhibit reverse transcriptase and also act as chain terminators because the lack of the 3' hydroxyl group prevents the formation of 3', 5' phosphodiester linkages in the DNA polymer. Ribavirin is a broad-spectrum antiviral agent whose mechanism of action involves interference with the formation of viral mRNA. There has been considerable controversy over the value of this drug in the treatment of HIV infection. Most investigators do not advocate its use. The interferons have a multiplicity of biochemical effects on cells, one of the net results of which is to render some cells resistant to infection with some viruses. Their use as a primary anti-HIV agent has been disappointing although there may be some role for the interferons in the management of Kaposi's sarcoma because of their anti-tumour properties.

21. TFTFT
The initial clinical trial of AZT was shown to reduce the morbidity and mortality associated with late-stage HIV infection. Surrogate markers of disease severity, such as CD4 cell count and p24 antigen levels, were also shown to improve in patients taking AZT. The latter findings have been reproduced in several trials, even in patients with asymptomatic infection. In the light of these encouraging findings in late-stage disease, it was hoped that the initiation of AZT therapy in asymptomatic anti-HIV-positive carriers would delay disease progression and enhance survival. Although short-term trials of AZT in asymptomatic patients did report promising results (e.g. a rise in CD4 count), the Anglo-French Concorde trial, the largest and longest one to date, failed to show any significant benefit in this group of patients in terms of survival or disease progression. This finding, incidentally, called into question the use of surrogate markers of disease severity as measurements of outcome, rather than defined morbidity or mortality. There have been independent trials of AZT plus acyclovir combination therapy purporting to show improved survival. The mechanisms underlying this effect are not clear. Both AZT and ganciclovir have toxic effects on the bone marrow, such that it is virtually impossible to treat patients with both drugs simultaneously. *In vitro* measurements of the sensitivity to AZT of isolates of HIV taken from the same patient before and 6 months after commencing AZT therapy, invariably demonstrate reduced sensitivity of the latter isolate in comparison with the former. This resistance is mediated by mutations in the reverse transcriptase gene, such that the enzyme is no longer able to recognize phosphorylated AZT. The clinical

significance of this resistance is hard to define. It may underlie the disappointing results of the early therapy trials referred to above because the earlier drug treatment is instituted the sooner resistant mutants will emerge.

Paper 9   Tropical viruses

1. FFTTT

See Table 9.1. Viruses such as measles and herpes simplex are, of course, as common in tropical climates as elsewhere. There are a number of viruses which are found mainly in such climates, however, and it is these that are referred to as 'tropical viruses' in this book. In turn, some of these may also be found outside tropical areas, a situation that has partly arisen from the ease of modern travel. The majority of tropical viruses are arthropod-borne.

Table 9.1 Epidemiology of commoner tropical viruses (also Table 3.2)

Virus family	Virus	Geographic distribution	Transmission
Arenaviridae	Lassa	W Africa	Rodents
	Junin	Argentina	Rodents
	Machupo	Bolivia	Rodents
Bunyaviridae	Bunyamwera	Uganda, SE Asia, S Africa, W Africa, C and S America USA, N Europe	Mosquito
	Phlebotomus	Mediterranean, Indian subcontinent	Phlebotomine
	Rift Valley	Africa	Mosquito
	Crimean–Congo haemorrhagic fever	Europe, Africa, C Asia, Middle East	Tick
	Hantaan	Europe, China, USA, Brazil, SE Asia	Rodents
	Oropouche	C and S America	Culicoides
	Bwamba	Africa	Mosquito
	Dugbe	Africa	Tick
	Bhaya	Africa, Europe, Asia	Tick
	Nairobi sheep disease	Africa, India	Tick
Filoviridae	Ebola	Sub-Saharan and E Africa	Infected humans
	Marburg	C and E Africa	Infected humans
Flaviviridae	Yellow fever	C and S America, Africa, W Indies	Mosquito

Table 9.1 cont.

Virus family	Virus	Geographic distribution	Transmission
Flaviviridae	Dengue	Pacific Islands, SE Asia, Australasia, Greece, Caribbean, C and S America, China, Nigeria	Mosquito
	Kyasanur Forest	India	Tick
	Kunjin	Australasia	Mosquito
	Omsk haemorrhagic fever	Former Soviet Union	Mosquito
	Zika	Africa, SE Asia	Mosquito
	Banzi	USA, W Indies	Mosquito
Orthomyxo-viridae	Thogoto	Africa, Europe	Tick
Reoviridae	Bluetongue	Worldwide	Culicoides
	Colorado tick	N America	Tick
Rhabdoviridae	Vesicular stomatitis virus	N and S America	Phlebotomine
	Chandipura	India, Africa	Phlebotomine
Togaviridae	Semliki forest	E and S Africa, SE Asia	Mosquito
	Sindbis	Egypt, India, S Africa Australia, N Europe	Mosquito
	Chikungunya	Africa, SE Asia	Mosquito
	Ross River	Australia	Mosquito
	O'nyong nyong	Africa	Mosquito
	Mayoro	S America	Mosquito
Unclassified	Quaranfil	Africa	Tick

2. TTTFT

See Table 9.2. The viruses most commonly associated with viral haemorrhagic fever are Lassa, Marburg, Ebola, dengue, yellow fever, Crimean-Congo haemorrhagic fever (CCHF) and Hantaan. The two Hantaan viruses, Hantaan and Puumula, cause haemorrhagic fever with renal syndrome (HFRS) which in different parts of the world is known as epidemic haemorrhagic fever, Korean haemorrhagic fever, nephropathia epidemica and haemorrhagic nephrosonephritis.

Table 9.2 Clinical features of commoner tropical viruses

Predominant clinical syndrome	Viruses
Fever	Dengue
	Banzi
	Zika
	Bunyamwera
	Nairobi sheep disease
	Dugbe
	Bluetongue
	Colorado tick
	Vesicular stomatitis
	Chandipura
	Quaranfil
Haemorrhagic fever	Dengue
	Yellow fever
	Lassa
	Ebola
	Marburg
	Junin
	Machupo
	Crimean–Congo haemorrhagic fever
	Rift Valley fever
	Omsk haemorrhagic fever
	Kyasanur forest
Haemorrhagic fever with renal syndrome	Hantaan
Arthritis/arthralgia	Chikungunya
	Mayoro
	O'nyong nyong
	Ross River
	Sindbis
Rash	Mayoro
	Sindbis
	Ross River
	Dengue
	Bwamba
Hepatitis	St. Louis encephalitis
	West Nile

3. TTTTT

Viral haemorrhagic fevers are so-called because they are associated with both fever and haemorrhage although frank bleeding does not occur in all cases. Fever is universal and other common features are hypovolaemia, proteinuria, lymphopenia, thrombocytopenia and platelet dysfunction and biochemical liver dysfunction with aspartate aminotransferase

Table 9.3 Clinical features of viral haemorrhagic fever syndromes

	Lassa	Ebola/Marburg	Dengue	Hantaan	CCHF	Junin/Machupo	Yellow fever
Incubation period	6–21 days	3–9 days (Marburg) 2–21 d (Ebola)	3–14 days	12–16 days	3–12 days	7–16 days	3–6 days
Reservoir	Multimammate mice	Unknown	Humans	Rodents	Hares, b'rds	Rodents, mice	Humans, primates
Oedema	Common	Uncommon	Common	Common	Uncommon	Common	Uncommon
Maculopapular rash	No	Common	Common	Common	Common	Common	No
Petechiae	No	Common	Common	Common	Common	Common	Common
Bleeding	15–20%	Common	Common	Uncommon	Common	Common	Common
Renal failure	With hypovolaemia	With hypovolaemia	With hypovolaemia	Majority	With hypovolaemia	With hypovolaemia	Common
Proteinuria	Uncommon	Common	Uncommon	Common	Uncommon	Uncommon	Common
Hepatic failure	Uncommon	Common	Uncommon	Uncommon	Common	Uncommon	Common
Encephalopathy	Common	Uncommon	Uncommon	Uncommon	Uncommon	Common	Uncommon
Other characteristic features	ECG changes in 70% Exudative pharyngitis Ataxia	Sore throat without exudate	Serous effusions	Facial erythema Palatal petechiae	Facial flushing Palatal petechiae	Tremor Strabismus	Bradycardia Jaundice
Case fatality (%)	15	50–90	1–5	1–10	5–20	15	1–5

levels raised more than alanine aminotransferase. General malaise, generalized pains and headaches are also common features. Hypovolaemic shock occurs in fatal cases. Adult respiratory distress occurs in severe cases of Lassa, dengue, Hantaan, Junin and Machupo. Other features are summarized in Table 9.3. The pathogenesis is complex but underlying the clinical manifestation is widespread organ damage.

4. TTTFT

Viral haemorrhagic fevers should be suspected on the basis of travel history and clinical features; exposure to rodents or arthropod vector may also be noted in the minority. Suspicion alone is often enough to institute isolation of the patient and barrier nursing; human-to-human transmission is uncommon but infected secretions pose a health hazard. Commoner diagnoses, in particular malaria, should initially be excluded. The differential diagnosis also includes rickettsial infection, typhoid, leptospirosis, relapsing fever, meningococcaemia, trypanosomiasis, measles, varicella, cytomegalovirus infection, drugs, thrombotic thrombocytopenic purpura and other collagen vascular disorders. Samples taken from the patient for any diagnosis should be discussed with the local pathology laboratory, preferably before being taken, to minimize the infectious risk. Specialist laboratories may have to be involved. Definitive diagnosis usually rests on specific antigen or antibody detection in serum (Table 9.4) although viruses can be found in other body fluids. Rapid diagnosis by detection of antigen or specific IgM is now used in many specialist laboratories. The management of the patient is

Table 9.4 Diagnostic tests used for viral haemorrhagic fevers

	Lassa	Ebola/ Marburg	Dengue	Hantaan	CCHF	Junin/ Machupo	Yellow fever
ELISA (IgM)	Yes	No	Yes	Yes	Yes	Yes	Yes
ELISA (Antigen detection)	Yes	No	Yes	No	Yes	Yes	Yes
Virus isolation	Blood, urine, throat	Blood	Blood	No	Blood	Blood	Blood
Fourfold IgG rise	Yes	Yes	Yes	Yes	Yes	Yes	Yes

supportive but ribavirin has been used successfully for Lassa fever, Rift Valley and Hantaan. Ribavirin has reduced the death rate of patients infected with Lassa virus from 57–67% to 5–9%. Oral ribavirin can also be given as prophylaxis for contacts. Blood and platelet trans-fusions, heparin, but not corticosteroids, may be indicated. Vaccines are only available against yellow fever.

Paper 10 Miscellaneous viruses and syndromes

EPSTEIN–BARR VIRUS

1. FTTTT

Epstein–Barr virus (EBV) is a member of the *Herpesviridae* (Table 7.1). It has the ability to infect lymphocytes and epithelial cells of genital and salivary origin. B lymphocytes tend to harbour latent virus in episomal form; the other cell types tend to be susceptible to lytic infection and shed virus. The virus is found worldwide and 80–90% of most populations studied have serological evidence of exposure to the virus by 5 years of age. This becomes almost 100% by 30 years of age. Transmission is predominantly by exchange of saliva from asymptomatic cases: 5–20% of healthy individuals shed the virus; over 65% of individuals with compromised cellular immunity. Transmission by sexual activity, blood transfusion and transplant tissue occurs but is relatively uncommon.

2. TTTFT

The majority of primary EBV infections are asymptomatic. In the immunocompetent, the commonest clinical manifestation is infectious mononucleosis (10.3). Over 90% of cases of this syndrome are caused by EBV. Other causes are cytomegalovirus, toxoplasmosis, human immunodeficiency virus and human herpesvirus-6. Complications such as aplastic anaemia may occur as part of this syndrome. EBV infection may cause lymphoproliferation in the immunosuppressed. Patients with X-linked lymphoproliferative syndrome (XLPS, also called Duncan's syndrome) have an abnormality of their X-chromosome so that they are unable, as an obvious manifestation, to synthesize gamma-interferon and have impaired cytotoxicity of lymphocytes. In boys with XLPS who suffer primary EBV infection, there is an inexorable expansion in EBV-infected B lymphocytes with hypogammaglobulinaemia, aplastic anaemia and lymphoproliferative malignancy. Over 60% die within 30 days; the survivors will usually die more slowly from lymphoma. This, and a non-familial sporadic form, are rare. In patients with acquired immunosuppression, particularly following transplantation, primary infection or reactivation of EBV can result in 'large-cell' lymphoproliferative disease. This occurs in 1–13% of patients post-renal transplantation. A mononucleosis-like syndrome is more common but less significant. In children with AIDS an unusual lymphoproliferative disorder, lymphocytic interstitial pneumonitis, occurs. In adults with AIDS, non-Hodgkin's lymphoma and oral hairy leukoplakia, which are more frequent than in the general population, are thought to be EBV-related. Other tumours associated with EBV infection are nasopharyngeal carcinoma, endemic Burkitt's lymphoma, Hodgkin's and non-Hodgkin's lymphoma. EBV is almost always found in these tumours but the precise role of EBV is unclear.

3. FTTTT
The incubation period of EBV-related infectious mononucleosis is 30–50 days. Onset is insidious with sore throat (75%), fever (95–100%) and lymphadenopathy (90–100%) in the majority of infected patients. General malaise, headache and splenomegaly also occur in the majority of patients. Less frequent clinical features are abdominal pain, chills, jaundice, periorbital oedema and rash. These occur in less than 25% of patients. The proportion of patients given ampicillin or amoxycillin who get a rash is however 100%; 25–50% of patients given other penicillins will also get a rash. The mechanism of this rash is unknown. Typically, the blood picture also shows abnormal lymphocytosis and heterophil antibodies.

4. TTTTT
Complications can occur before, during or after the mononucleosis illness (Table 10.1). Depression and/or lethargy are the commonest. Most are uncommon or rare.

Table 10.1 Complications of infectious mononucleosis

System	Complication	Comments
Haematological	Haemolytic anaemia	Occurs in 0.5–3%, resolves spontaneously
	Thrombocytopenia	Occurs in up to 50%, resolves spontaneously
	Platelet dysfunction	Resolves spontaneously
	Agranulocytosis	Rare, resolves spontaneously
	Aplastic anaemia	Rare, may be fatal
	Splenic rupture	May follow minor trauma Most cases survive with intervention
Neurological	Encephalitis	Uncommon
	Aseptic meningitis	Uncommon
	Seizures	Uncommon
	Guillain–Barré syndrome	Uncommon
	Optic neuritis	Uncommon
	Cranial neuropathies	Uncommon
	Peripheral neuropathy	Uncommon

Table 10.1 cont.

System	Complication	Comments
Neurological	Subacute sclerosing Panencephalitis	Uncommon
Psychiatric	Depression	Common
	Psychosis	Rare
Respiratory	Pharyngeal lymphoid hyperplasia	Occurs in less than 1%, may lead to obstruction
	Pneumonia	Rare clinically, 15% of all cases have X-ray changes
	Pleural effusion	
	Secondary streptococcal pharyngitis	
Cardiac	ECG abnormalities	Occur in 6%, may be fatal
	Myocarditis	
	Pericarditis	
Hepatobiliary	Hepatitis	Most patients have abnormal liver function biochemically, 5–10% will be jaundiced
	Reye's syndrome	Rare
	Pancreatitis	Rare, usually self-limiting
	Mesenteric lymphadenopathy	May be mistaken for appendicitis
Renal	Glomerulonephritis	Rare
	Haemolytic-uraemic syndrome	Rare
	Renal osteodystrophy	Rare
Others	Orchitis	Occurs in 10–20%
	Myalgia	
	Arthritis	Very rare
	Conjunctivitis	Very rare
	Papilloedema	Very rare
	Death	Occurs in 1 in 3000
	Persistent mononucleosis	Infectious mononucleosis lasting 12 months or more occurs in less than 5%

5. FTTTT

Non-specific and specific tests are to confirm the diagnosis of EBV infection. Heterophil antibodies are IgM antibodies that are induced by EBV (and other agents) that are not specific for the eliciting agent. The Paul–Bunnell and Monospot tests are means of detecting these and are considered positive at titres of 1:16 and 1:2, respectively.

Heterophil antibody is usually detectable at the onset of clinical illness but may occasionally take up to 4 weeks to develop. The Paul–Bunnell test is the more sensitive and is positive in 70–90% of cases whereas 50% of children under the age of 5 years may be negative by the Monospot test. It is however clear that specific tests are not necessary in the majority of cases of infectious mononucleosis. Specific serology relies on the detection of antibodies to three groups of viral antigens: early antigens (EA), nuclear antigens (NA) and capsid antigens (VCA) (Table 10.2). There are two components of the early antigens: restricted (EA-R) and diffuse (EA-D). Burkitt's lymphoma is characteristically associated with IgG anti-EA-R. Infectious mononucleosis and nasopharyngeal carcinoma are associated with IgG anti-EA-D. Detection of EBV-specific IgA in saliva is suggestive of nasopharyngeal carcinoma.

Table 10.2 Serological tests used to diagnose EBV infection

	Current infection	*Recent infection*	*Past infection*
Heterophil antibodies	+	±	Rare
IgM anti-VCA	+	±	−
IgG anti-VCA	+	+	+
IgG anti-EA	+	±	−
IgG anti-EBNA	±	±	+

6. TFFFF

Uncomplicated infectious mononucleosis is a self-limiting disease and rarely requires more than analgesics for sore throat. Lymphoproliferative disease in the immunocompromised patient is generally managed with either withdrawal or reduction of immunosuppressive agents but a high failure rate is common. Anecdotal reports of successful use of ganciclovir, acyclovir, methisazone, recombinant alpha-interferon, anti-B lymphocyte monoclonal antibody and metronidazole have been reported. In many of these instances spontaneous regression may have occurred. Acyclovir appears to be of benefit in the management of oral hairy leukoplakia. No vaccines have yet been made commercially available but a number are undergoing clinical trials.

CYTOMEGALOVIRUS

7. TTTTT

Cytomegalovirus (CMV) shares the physical properties of other herpesviruses. It also exhibits latency and despite the lack of a specifically associated malignancy, it has oncogenic properties. Antigenic heterogeneity is well recognized although a universal typing system has not been developed. The virus gets its name from the characteristic swollen cells that it produces in cell culture. The virus is found worldwide and over 40% of people in developed countries (over 90% in developing countries) acquire the virus. The highest rate of acquisition is in the first year of life. Poorer socioeconomic conditions and sexual promiscuity lead to higher prevalence ratios than the general population; CMV is found in practically all AIDS patients. Transmission can occur by a variety of routes: *in utero*, perinatal, close contact, by blood transfusion and sexually. The virus can be found in urine, saliva and other bodily secretions. Ten per cent of non-pregnant women shed the virus from their cervix at any one time, 10–30% of children in their urine and 5–15% of adults in pharyngeal secretions. Virus is also found in faeces, breast milk, tears and target organs.

8. TTTTT
The vast majority of CMV infections in the immunocompetent adult are asymptomatic. The commonest clinical manifestation is fever

Table 10.3 Clinical manifestations of infection with CMV

System	Manifestation	Comments
General	Infectious mononucleosis	Heterophil antibody-negative (CMV causes 50% of such cases) Affects mainly adults
	Post-perfusion syndrome	Mononucleosis occurring several weeks to months after blood transfusion Infection may be primary, reactivation or reinfection
Hepatobiliary	Hepatitis	Uncommon, occurs more commonly post-transfusion, spontaneous recovery
	Pancreatitis	Uncommon
Respiratory	Pneumonia	Uncommon except in immuno-compromised and infants, may be asymptomatic, self-limiting in immunocompetent, high mortality in immunocompromised
Eye	Chorioretinitis	occurs in 4% of immuno-compromised, 50% of these will have unilateral involvement, 50% will progress to partial or total visual impairment

Table 10.3 Contd

System	Manifestation	Comments
	Conjunctivitis	Uncommon
	Uveitis	Rare
	Iritis	Rare
	Cataract	Rare
	Optic neuropathy	Rare
	Microphthalmia	Rare
Gastrointestinal	Oesophagitis	Uncommon except in immuno-compromised, can lead to haemorrhage
	Gastritis	Uncommon except in immuno-compromised, can lead to haemorrhage
	Colitis	Uncommon except in immuno-compromised, can lead to haemorrhage
	Proctitis	Uncommon except in immuno-compromised, can lead to haemorrhage
Neurological	Meningoencephalitis	Rare except in immuno-compromised
	Encephalitis	Usually diagnosed post mortem in immunocompromised
	Polyneuritis	Uncommon but occurs in immunocompromised
	Guillain–Barré syndrome	Rare
Haematological	Thrombocytopenic purpura	Good prognosis
	Haemolytic anaemia	Death uncommon, spontaneous resolution
	Vasculitis and disseminated intravascular coagulation	Rare
	Leukopenia	
Others	Acute pericarditis	Rare
	Myocarditis	Rare, may be fatal
	Arthritis	Uncommon
	Cystitis	Uncommon
	Glomerulonephritis	Rare

either alone or as part of a mononucleosis syndrome. Other illnesses are less common except in the immunocompromised (Table 10.3). Fever and pneumonia are common illnesses caused by CMV in post-transplant patients. Pneumonia, oesophagitis, colitis, chorioretinitis and encephalitis are common in patients with AIDS. Disease can occur as a result of both primary infection and reactivation of latent virus.

9. TTTFT

Neonatal infection with CMV is common: approximately 0.5–2.5% of neonates have CMV viruria; 5–10% of these will have symptomatic disease at birth; one-third of these will die and most of the rest will have permanent neurological damage. Symptomatic infection from *in utero* transmission is almost always due to primary infection in the mother although, conversely, only 15% of primary maternal infections will result in cytomegalic inclusion disease (CID). Perinatal infection may present weeks after birth and affect about 10% of infants. Most cases are symptomatic but some may develop pneumonitis. The clinical spectrum of CID includes hepatosplenomegaly, jaundice, petechiae, microcephaly, deafness, chorioretinitis and neuromuscular disorders as common features. Pneumonia may also occur and is often a marker of more severe disease. Chronic sequelae are common and include tooth defects in 40%, neurological damage (hearing deficit, mental retardation, microcephaly) and chronic liver disease. Investigations reveal atypical lymphocytosis, thrombocytopenia and abnormal liver function tests in the majority. Chest X-ray changes, including calcification, may also be noted.

10. TFTTT

The standard means for confirming infection with CMV is culture from urine of the virus in cell monolayers. It may take up to 21 days or more before cytopathic effects are noted. Virus can also be isolated from other specimens such as bronchoalveolar lavage fluid, saliva, throat swabs, semen, buffy coat, cervical mucus and infected biopsy material. The delay in diagnosis by culture is unhelpful if therapy is contemplated and the process is often made more rapid by the detection of early viral antigens in cultures by fluorescence labelled antibodies (DEAFF test). This can shorten diagnosis to 24 hours. There have been many modifications of this method, some of which enable even more rapid diagnosis. In specimens with adequate cellular material it may be possible to detect viral antigens directly or observe characteristic 'owl's eye' intranuclear inclusions with Wright–Giemsa staining. The former has a sensitivity compared with culture of 80–90%, the latter less than 75%. Detection of a fourfold rise in CMV-specific IgG also confirms acute infection. This has been shown to be more sensitive than virus isolation if the later samples are collected at 2, 4 and 8 weeks after acute illness. Many test formats are used but the most sensitive are based on ELISA or RIA. Tests for CMV-specific IgM are now commercially available and should prove to be particularly useful in the diagnosis of neonatal infection. Electron microscopy of urine from patients with CID is occasionally useful. Gene detection methods are also widely available but are not routinely used. Interpretation of tests is summarized in Table 10.4. Caution should be taken when considering whether clinical disease is due to active infection with cytomegalovirus: some tests such as detection of the virus in peripheral blood are more helpful than others as indicators of disease causation.

Table 10.4 Diagnostic tests used in CMV infection

	Culture	*IgG antibody*	*IgM antibody*	*Cytology*
CID	+ within 2 weeks of birth (urine, saliva)	+ (if negative rules out diagnosis)	±	+
Perinatal	+ negative at birth (urine, saliva)	+	±	±
Adult	+ (urine, others)	+ (fourfold rise)	+	±
Immuno- compromised	+ (urine, others)	+ (± by CFT)	+	±

11. FTTTT

CMV infection does not need specific treatment except in those with severe disease or in the immunocompromised who are at risk of developing severe disease. The first measure in this latter group is withdrawal or reduction of immunosuppressive therapy if possible. If this is ineffective or not possible then ganciclovir is the current drug of choice. The drug alone or in combination with CMV hyperimmune globulin or foscarnet has been used for treating severe CMV disease. The use of anti-CMV monoclonal antibodies is also under investigation. Ganciclovir appears to be more effective in treating chorioretinitis and gastrointestinal infection than pneumonia; an explanation for this is that the latter may be an immunopathological condition. Relapse of disease is common after cessation of ganciclovir if the patient remains immunosuppressed. Disease also often progresses on treatment. Foscarnet has a similar success rate to ganciclovir but has a particular role after treatment failure with ganciclovir or in combination with it. Both drugs are toxic. Ganciclovir is frequently associated with bone marrow suppression and with abnormal liver function tests, fever, rash and CNS disorders (anxiety, drowsiness, fits, etc.). The most severe adverse effect of foscarnet is dose-dependent nephrotoxicity. Metabolic abnormalities such as hypocalcaemia (occasionally fatal), hyper-phosphataemia, hypokalaemia, hypomagnesaemia and nephrogenic diabetes insipidus are also not uncommon. Penile ulceration is a peculiar effect of foscarnet therapy in some patients. Prevention of CMV infection is perhaps more important. Principles of this include the following. (1) Testing of both donors and recipients for CMV status. Ideally seronegative patients receive only seronegative blood and blood products. If this is not possible then administration of anti-CMV immunoglobulin has been shown to decrease the likelihood of CMV disease. Prophylactic anti-CMV immunoglobulin in seropositive patients is also under con-sideration. (2) Monitoring of immunosuppressed patients at regular intervals (weekly in some centres) for CMV infection. This is usually post-transplantation as immunosuppression is temporary. It is not cost-effective in patients with progressive immunodeficiencies, e.g. AIDS. There are a number of further strategies under investigation that may also reduce the incidence of CMV disease in transplant patients. (3) Immunization with live attenuated Towne vaccine has been shown to reduce the severity of CMV disease in seronegative patients who receive organs from seropositive patients. It does not reduce the rate of infection. (4) Filtering blood products before administration has been shown to reduce the load of CMV-infected cells. (5) The role of antiviral prophylaxis is as yet unclear although acyclovir prophylaxis in renal transplant patients and ganciclovir prophylaxis in bone marrow transplant patients is used.

VIRUSES AND CANCER

12. TFTTF

The pathogenesis of malignancy is complex but is usually as a result of genetic changes in host DNA so that control of cell proliferation is lost. African Burkitt's lymphoma is an example of a genetic aberration (translocation of part of chromosome 8 to chromosome 14, 2 or 22) which results in the over-production of a cellular oncogene, c-myc. Epstein–Barr virus also appears to be involved. It is known to be able to immortalize cells *in vitro* and is always present in these tumours. Other cofactors, such as concurrent malarial infection, also appear to play a role. Other malignancies where viruses are thought to be important in causation are primary hepatocellular carcinoma (hepatitis B and hepatitis C), nasopharyngeal carcinoma (EBV), adult T cell leukaemia (HTLV-1) and cervical cancer (human papillomavirus). There have been reports of a putative herpesvirus, Inoue–Melnick virus, found in cases of colonic carcinoma but a very strong genetic predisposition appears to be the key factor.

13. TTTTF
Screening of cancer patients for antiviral antibodies is useful for assessing the risk of reactivation of latent virus which may cause serious disease and/or susceptibility to primary disease which may have a serious outcome. The herpesviruses (and polyomaviruses) are the viruses that fall into the first category. Potentially most viruses fall into the latter group but particularly measles virus in children is of potential concern. As many patients receive blood transfusions, there is also an argument for regular screening for hepatitis B, hepatitis C and human immunodeficiency virus, although the last of these has other connotations.

APLASTIC ANAEMIA AND THROMBOCYTOPENIA

14. TTTFT
Other viruses commonly associated are HIV and hepatitis C virus. Less common are hepatitis A and hepatitis B virus. B19, dengue and EBV have been shown to be able to infect haematopoietic cells; the mechanisms by which the other viruses cause aplasia are unclear.

15. TFTTT
Other viruses associated are cytomegalovirus, rubella and human immunodeficiency virus. The mechanism by which thrombocytopenia is produced is usually uncertain.

CONGENITAL INFECTIONS

16. TTTFT
A 'TORCH' screen has been habitually requested in the UK for the diagnosis of congenital infection. This is an acronym for toxoplasmosis, rubella, cytomegalovirus and herpes simplex. Serological tests to determine the presence of antibody to these agents are used. Most such screens are unhelpful and it is better to clinically

assess the likelihood of specific infections and request appropriate investigations.

CONJUNCTIVITIS AND KERATITIS

17. TTTTF
Viruses cause up to 20% of cases of non-epidemic conjunctivitis in children and 14% of adult cases. The clinical syndrome is one of a self-limiting illness with watery discharge. There may be mild itching and preauricular lymphadenopathy. There may also be a concomitant upper respiratory tract illness. Adenoviruses and enteroviruses are the commonest agents associated with epidemic conjunctivitis as well as being common in non-epidemic cases. Apart from herpes simplex, adenoviruses and enteroviruses, sporadic cases may be due to EBV, VZV, papillomaviruses, influenza, measles, mumps and molluscum contagiosum. There are usually features of infection with these agents elsewhere on the body.

18. TTTFT
The most severe form of viral keratitis is that due to herpes simplex viruses, particularly if it occurs in the perinatal period. Approximately 40% will recur. Dendritic or geographic corneal ulceration is characteristic with spontaneous resolution within 2 weeks in 80%. The others may have scarring without topical acyclovir therapy. Steroids are contraindicated as virus replication is enhanced. Epidemic kerato-conjunctivitis due to adenoviruses has a characteristic clinical picture of corneal opacities which resolve in 2–3 weeks. Topical corticosteroids enhance resolution which suggests that direct viral infection is not responsible. Ten per cent of patients with herpes zoster will have the ophthalmic division of the trigeminal nerve affected. Oral acyclovir is the treatment of choice. Ocular infection is also an unusual complication of primary chickenpox. Rarer causes of keratitis are vaccinia (by auto-inoculation), measles (rarely causes blindness unless the patient is malnourished) and EBV. HIV can be detected in corneal epithelium but does not appear to be a clinical problem.

MYOCARDITIS

19. TTTTT
See Table 10.5. Enteroviruses are responsible for 50% of cases with a defined viral aetiology. Diagnosis is made on clinical grounds with

laboratory identification of a specific virus. There is no specific treatment although ribavirin has shown promise in murine enteroviral myocarditis.

Table 10.5 Viral causes of myocarditis

Common causes	Less common causes
Enteroviruses (particularly Coxsackie B)	Rabies
Mumps	Hepatitis B
Influenza	Rubella
Measles	Dengue
	Adenoviruses
	Varicella-zoster
	Epstein–Barr
	Cytomegalovirus
	Vaccinia
	Yellow fever
	Viral haemorrhagic fever viruses

ARTHRITIS

20. TTTTF

The viruses most commonly associated with arthritis are rubella, B19 and mumps. It also occurs in association with urticaria as an immune-complex phenomenon with hepatitis B infection. Ross River virus has been a frequent cause in Australasia. It is also a prominent feature of other alphavirus infections: O'nyong nyong, Chikungunya and Sindbis. Rarely associated are vaccinia, adenoviruses, EBV, VZV, influenza and lymphocytic choriomeningitis virus. Whether these viruses cause arthritis is doubtful.

MISCELLANEOUS

21. TTTFT

Both CMV and HSV-1 have been found in atherosclerotic plaques and there is a sero-epidemiological association. Moreover, a chicken herpesvirus, Marek's disease virus, causes atherosclerotic plaques in chickens which can be prevented by immunization against the virus. The majority of patients with acquired porphyria cutanea tarda have evidence of hepatitis C infection. Particles with characteristic herpesvirus morphology have been seen in patients with meningioma. This virus is called Inoue–Melnick after its co-discoverers but both the virus and disease association require substantiation. CMV infection is uncommonly complicated by vasculitis.

22. TTTTT

See Table 10.6. The clinical significance of these antibodies is unclear.

Table 10.6 Autoantibodies arising from viral infections

Virus	Autoantibodies
Coxsackie B	Cardiac muscle
Cytomegalovirus	DNA, erythrocytes, immunoglobulin, lymphocytes, neutrophils, platelets, smooth muscle
Epstein–Barr	DNA, cytoskeleton, erythrocytes, lymphocytes, neutrophils, platelets, smooth muscle, thyroglobulin
Hepatitis B	DNA, immunoglobulins, lymphocytes, neutrophils, platelets
Hepatitis C	DNA, immunoglobulins
Human immunodeficiency	DNA, erythrocytes, immunoglobulin, lymphocytes, neutrophils, platelets
Mumps	Cardiac muscle, DNA, cytoskeleton, insulin, lymphocytes, pancreatic islet cells
Varicella-zoster	Cytoskeleton, insulin

Paper 11   Antiviral agents and prophylaxis

ANTIVIRAL DRUGS

1. TFTFT
There are few licensed antiviral drugs compared with the plethora of antibacterial agents (Table 11.1). These are all virustatic. Exogenous interferon (IFN) was the first agent used specifically as an antiviral. Because of the role of endogenous interferon it was hoped that it would have a broad spectrum of activity. This did not turn out to be feasible and IFN currently has a place only in the management of chronic hepatitis B, chronic hepatitis C and warts. Fucidin was reported to have a beneficial effect in patients with HIV but this has been shown not to be because of any antiviral activity of the drug. Heparin analogues are under investigation as anti-HIV agents but none has been licensed.

Table 11.1 Mechanism of action of antiviral drugs

Drug	Mechanism(s) of action
Acyclovir	Nucleoside analogue, inhibits nucleic acid synthesis; active form produced by viral thymidine kinase
Ribavirin	Nucleoside analogue, inhibits nucleic acid synthesis, possibly by inhibiting viral RNA polymerase
Amantadine Rimantadine	Inhibit virus uncoating, maturation and egress from cell
Ganciclovir	Nucleoside analogue, blocks nucleic acid synthesis by inhibiting viral thymidine kinase and other enzymes
Azidothymidine Dideoxyinosine Dideoxycytidine	Nucleoside analogues, inhibits nucleic acid synthesis by inhibition of reverse transcriptase
Foscarnet	Blocks protein synthesis by inhibition of RNA and DNA polymerases
Idoxuridine	Nucleoside analogue, inhibits DNA synthesis
Vidarabine	Nucleoside analogue, blocks DNA synthesis by inhibiting DNA polymerases

2. TFFTT
See Table 11.1.

3. FTFTT
See Table 11.2.

Table 11.2 Indications for currently available antiviral agents

Drug	Route of administration	Indications
Acyclovir	Oral	Severe primary genital herpes
		Severe or frequent (six or more recurrences) genital and oral herpes
		Suppression of frequent (six or more recurrences) of genital herpes
		Suppression of mucocutaneous herpes in immunocompromised
		Treatment of mucocutaneous herpes in immunocompromised
		Zoster infection in immunocompromised
		Ophthalmic zoster
		Hairy leukoplakia in AIDS patients
	Intravenous	Herpes encephalitis
		Neonatal herpes
		Severe genital herpes
		Severe herpes simplex infection in immunocompromised
		Severe varicella-zoster in immunocompetent
		Varicella-zoster in immunocompromised
	Topical	Herpes keratitis
		Possibly primary genital herpes
		Possibly frequent genital herpes
Ganciclovir	Intravenous	CMV retinitis in immunocompromised
		CMV pneumonia in immunocompromised
Amantadine/ Rimantadine	Oral	Influenza A treatment and prophylaxis
Ribavirin	Aerosol	Severe RSV infection
	Intravenous	Lassa fever and other viral haemorrhagic fevers
	Oral	Prophylaxis of contacts of Lassa fever and other viral haemorrhagic fevers
Azidothymidine	Oral	Symptomatic HIV infection
Dideoxyinosine/ Dideoxycytidine	Oral	Intolerance or failure of azidothymidine
Foscarnet	Intravenous	CMV retinitis
		Acyclovir-resistant HSV or VZV
Idoxuridine	Topical	Herpes labialis
Vidarabine	Topical	Herpes keratitis
	Intravenous	Herpes encephalitis
		Neonatal herpes

4. TTFTT

See Table 11.3. Unwanted effects may be more common with combination therapy although unlike the use of antibiotics such therapy is unusual. An exception is the management of AIDS where azidothymidine (AZT) and other antivirals may be required. The additive bone marrow toxicity of ganciclovir precludes its simultaneous use with AZT, an indication for foscarnet. Potential beneficial effects of combination therapy, e.g. AZT and ddI, are under investigation.

Table 11.3 Adverse effects of antiviral drugs

Drug	Common adverse effects	Less common adverse effects
Acyclovir	None	Renal impairment (in dehydrated) Rashes Gastrointestinal intolerance Emergence of drug-resistant strains
Ganciclovir	Reversible bone marrow suppression in 25%	Potentially teratogenic Renal impairment Abnormal liver function Fever Rash
Amantadine	Insomnia Nausea Vestibulitis	
Rimantadine	Drug-resistant strains in 50% of patients on 6 days or more of treatment	As for amantadine but less frequent
Ribavirin	Anaemia Teratogenicity	Potentially immunosuppressive
Azidothymidine	Bone marrow suppression Nausea Headache Drug-resistance	Myopathy Renal impairment
Dideoxyinosine	Painful peripheral neuropathy Pancreatitis Diarrhoea	
Dideoxycytidine	Peripheral neuropathy	
Idoxuridine	None from topical use	
Vidarabine	Nausea/vomiting Megaloblastosis Myoclonus Myopathy	
Foscarnet	Renal impairment	Genital ulcer Bone marrow suppression

5. TTTTT

Antiviral resistance occurs either as therapeutic resistance because the drug cannot achieve high enough local concentrations or because of genetic mutation in the virus. Acyclovir-resistant herpesviruses are being found more frequently in immunosuppressed patients but in general are less virulent except in those with severe immunosuppression. Sensitive strains may again predominate if acyclovir is withdrawn. Alternatively, foscarnet can be used as it has a different mechanism of action. Rimantidine-resistant influenza A strains appear to be pathogenic and amantadine does not appear to be an alternative as it has the same mechanism of action. Detection of drug-resistant strains can be made by culture *in vitro* but not all viruses or strains are easily cultivable. Moreover, minority sensitive strains may still grow more easily than the resistant strains. Direct detection of mutants by polymerase chain reaction (PCR) offers a more reliable method in those viruses where the mutation conferring drug resistance is known.

VIRAL VACCINES AND IMMUNOPROPHYLAXIS

6. TTTTT

Vaccination against viruses has reduced dramatically the incidence of those diseases that have been targeted. For full efficacy and maximum uptake, some general principles are applied. (1) Consent of the patient should be noted, not necessarily written. (2) The vaccine should be kept, reconstituted, administered and used within the date recommended by the manufacturer. If the vaccine is sent by post, it should be under conditions appropriate for the vaccine. (3) If the prospective vaccinee is suffering from an acute febrile illness then the vaccination should be postponed until the patient has recovered. (4) Alcohol can inactivate live vaccines so if used as a skin preparation it should be allowed to evaporate before administration of the vaccine. (5) Live virus vaccines should be given at a different site or time from human normal immunoglobulin (HNIG) as the latter may interfere with the efficacy of the former. If HNIG has already been given, a gap of 3 months is preferred before administering the live vaccine. The principal exception is yellow fever vaccine administered in non-endemic areas where HNIG is unlikely to contain yellow fever antibodies. (6) Contraindications to vaccine use should be noted (11.7).

11.7 TTTTF

Apart from those listed, a previous history of generalized reaction to a vaccine component is a contraindication. The following constitute a general reaction: fever of 39.5°C or greater within 48 hours of vaccination that is not attributable to other causes, anaphylaxis, bronchospasm, laryngeal oedema, collapse, convulsions or encephalopathy. These contraindications are not absolute and vaccine may still be used if the risks of disease outweigh those of the vaccine. Previous history of illness, family history of adverse reaction, family history of neurological disease, contact with infectious disease, atopy *per se* (hayfever, asthma, eczema), treatment with local steroids, prematurity, HIV infection without overt immunosuppression and pregnancy in the vaccinee's mother are not contraindications. There are a few exceptions to these general rules, e.g. MMR vaccine can be given to HIV-positive individuals. Contraindications to inactivated vaccines are few, principally a history of previous severe adverse reaction.

8. FTTTF
See Table 11.4. Viral vaccines are live attenuated strains, inactivated virus or purified antigens (recombinant or otherwise). Because of local replication, live strains tend to produce a superior immune response in terms of both the antibody levels and the duration of immunity. The principal disadvantages of such vaccines are that they are more likely to produce clinical disease, particularly if they mutate to a virulent strain, as has occurred with polio vaccines.

Table 11.4 Currently available viral vaccines in the UK

Vaccine	Live?	Conditions of administration	Specific unwanted effects
Poliomyelitis (Sabin)	Yes Trivalent	Oral Primary course at 2, 3, 4 months of age Boosters at 4–5 years and 15–18 years of age Boosters to travellers to endemic areas	Poliomyelitis (0.5–1/ million vials used)
Poliomyelitis (Salk)	No Trivalent	As above but to immunocom- promised. Given sc or im	
Measles	Yes	Now given as MMR	Acute febrile convulsions (1 per 1000 cases) Rash and fever Inhibits response to tuberculin Can exacerbate TB

Table 11.4 Contd

Vaccine	Live?	Conditions of administration	Specific unwanted effects
Mumps	Yes	Now given as MMR	Parotid swelling (1 per 1000 cases) Meningoencephalitis (up to 1 per 10 000 cases)
Rubella	Yes	Now given as MMR	Thrombocytopenia Arthralgia/arthritis
MMR	Yes	Given im or deep sc at 12–18 months of age	As for individual components
Influenza	No Trivalent (2 strains of flu A, and 1 of flu B)	Given im or sc Single dose in elderly, two doses in children Given to 'at risk' patients before epidemics	30% vaccine failure
Hepatitis B	No Recombinant	Given im or sc Primary course at 0.1, 6 months Given to 'high risk' groups	5–10% poor response Uncommonly, flu-like illness, rash, arthropathy and abnormal liver function
Hepatitis A	No	Given im as 2 doses 2–4 weeks apart Given to travellers to endemic areas and sewerage workers	Uncommon
Rabies	No	Given as deep sc, im or id Can be given pre- or post-exposure	Neomycin sensitivity
Yellow fever	Yes	Given deep sc Given to laboratory workers and travellers	5–10% have mild headache and flu-like illness Short-lived encephalitis
Japanese B encephalitis	No	Given sc, 3 doses at 0, 7–14 and 28 days Given to travellers to endemic areas	None specific
Tick-borne encephalitis	No	Given in, 3 doses at 0, 1 week and 1 year	None specific Not licensed

Table 11.4 Contd

Vaccine	Live?	Conditions of administration	Specific unwanted effects
		Given to long-term travellers to endemic areas	
Varicella-zoster	Yes	Given im to immunocompro-mised patients	Uncommonly, fever and rash Not licensed
Vaccinia	Yes	Given sc to laboratory workers	Encephalitis (rare) Vaccinia Eczema vaccinatum

im, intramuscular; sc, subcutaneous

Further reading

The following references have been used in the preparation of this book and are recommended further reading:

Belshe, R.B. (ed.) (1991) *Textbook of Human Virology*, Mosby, St. Louis, USA.

Benenson, A.S. (ed.) (1990) *Control of Communicable Diseases in Man*, Washington, USA.

Department of Health (1992) *Immunisation Against Infectious Disease*, HMSO, London, England.

White, D.O. and Fenner, F.J. (1986) *Medical Virology*, Academic Press, Orlando, USA.

Zuckerman, A.J., Banatvala, J.E. and Pattison, J.R. (eds) (1990) *Principles and Practice of Clinical Virology*, John Wiley, Chichester, England.

Appendix:
commonly used abbreviations

ADCC	Antibody-dependent cellular cytotoxicity
AIDS	Acquired immunodeficiency syndrome
AZT	Azidothymidine
CAT	Computer-aided tomography
CCHF	Crimean–Congo haemorrhagic fever
CDC	Center for Disease Control (Atlanta, Georgia, USA)
CFT	Complement fixation test
CID	Cytomegalic inclusion disease
cm	Centimetre
CMV	Cytomegalovirus
CT	Computerized tomography
CTL	Cytotoxic T cell
DNA	Deoxyribonucleic acid
EBV	Epstein–Barr virus
EEG	Electroencephalography
ELISA	Enzyme-linked immunosorbent
EM	Electron microscopy
HAI	Haemagglutination-inhibition
HCW	Healthcare worker
HIV	Human immunodeficiency virus
HSV	Herpes simplex virus
id	intradermal
im	intramuscular
iv	intravenous
kb	kilobase(s)
MAC	*Mycobacterium avium-intracellulare* complex
mm	millimetre
nm	nanometre
PCP	*Pneumocystis carinii* pneumonia
PCR	Polymerase chain reaction
ppm	parts per million
RIA	Radioimmunoassay
RNA	Ribonucleic acid
RSV	Respiratory syncytial virus
VZV	Varicella-zoster virus

Index